HOMOEOPATHY

Beth MacEoin

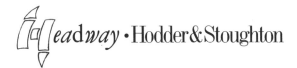

Headway · Hodder & Stoughton

The publishers would like to thank the following for giving permission to reproduce copyright photographic material in this book; p9/10, Hahnemann Society, London; p17, Chris Day, Alternative Veterinary Medicine Centre, Faringdon, Oxon; p42, Bart's Medical Picture Library; p44, British Dental Association; p49, Bart's Medical Picture Library; p62, David Woodfall/NHPA; p64, J Allan Cash Photolibrary; p73, J Allan Cash Photolibrary; p94, Bart's Medical Picture Library; p110, Hulton Deutsch Collection Ltd. Commissioned photographs by Roddy Paine.

British Library Cataloguing in Publication Data

MacEoin, Beth
  Homoeopathy. – (Headway Lifeguides
  Series)
  I. Title II. Series
  615.5

  ISBN 0–340–56578–0

First published 1992

Typeset by Wearset, Boldon, Tyne and Wear
Printed in Great Britain for the educational publishing division of Hodder & Stoughton Ltd, Mill Road, Dunton Green, Sevenoaks, Kent by Thomson Litho Ltd.

For Denis, without whose patience, love, and encouragement this book would never have been written.

ACKNOWLEDGEMENTS

My warmest thanks are due to many people who have offered help and advice with this project. At the earliest stage my agent Teresa Chris offered immensely practical help and encouragement, for which I shall always be grateful to her. Jayne Booth was a delight to work with as an editor, as well as offering pertinent advice when needed.

Thanks must be extended to Stephen Gordon, who has been especially helpful in offering advice on the more technical aspects of this manuscript. I am also deeply indebted to John Tomlinson, not just for his reading of the manuscript at an early stage, but also for his hospitality and patience during the photo shoot at Helios pharmacy. Angela Morse must also be thanked, not only for her incisive comments and advice on the text of this book, but for initially encouraging in me a love of this subject. Rima Handley must also not be forgotten for having taken time out from an already extremely busy schedule to read the manuscript. Thanks must also be extended to Dana Ullman and Stephen Cummings, whose book on the same subject provided me with inspiration, and some very practical advice on the nuts and bolts of first aid.

My mother Nancy must also be thanked for keeping the household sane while I have been occupied with writing this book. Finally, the largest measure of thanks must go to Denis, Daniel, and Jonathan. Without their unwavering vision and enthusiasm for this project I would have given up in despair and impatience many times.

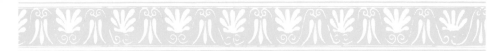

CONTENTS

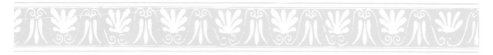

FOREWORD

Homoeopathy is one of the most effective forms of medicine that has ever been discovered. However its enormous powers are appreciated by relatively few since it has been overshadowed by the monolithic structures of orthodox medicine. As the twentieth century draws to its close the world has become a little more sceptical of the claims of the drug companies and a little more careful of the pollution that drugs bring to the planet. It may be that homoeopathy's time has come at last.

This is a clear and concise introduction to the fascinating subject of homoeopathy written by a practising homoeopath. It contains a good deal of helpful advice about the treatment of a variety of simple illnesses and guides the reader carefully through the process of selecting homoeopathic remedies for many of the common conditions that may be met with in the home and family. It contains helpful tables which simplify the selection process while at the same time leading the reader to prescribe in the most holistic way possible.

RIMA HANDLEY, M.A., D. Phil., F.S. Hom.
Dean, Northern College of Homoeopathic Medicine

INTRODUCTION

This book is intended as basic introduction to homoeopathy for the person who knows nothing about the subject, as well as providing a very practical self-help handbook which may be used for those conditions that can be safely managed at home. As always in a book of this kind, very firm guidelines are given about when to call for professional help, and symptoms that indicate you are likely to be getting out of your depth are highlighted. (In severe emergencies, your first port of call should, of course, be your GP or the emergency department of your local hospital. In less pressing circumstances, existing patients of a professional or doctor homoeopath will have first recourse to their practitioner. Individuals without a homoeopath should contact their GP initially, and when the immediate emergency has been taken care of, may consider finding a competent homoeopath to investigate the problem more deeply.) However, I am sure you will find judicious homoeopathic prescribing within this framework a rewarding, exciting and enjoyable experience, even if the challenge seems rather daunting at first.

What is homoeopathic medicine?

Homoeopathic medicine is a system of healing which has been in existence for almost 200 years. It is practised by both orthodoxly trained doctors and professional homoeopaths on a world-wide basis. In expert hands, homoeopathy provides a way of restoring the sick individual to good health in a gentle, thorough, and effective manner.

The concept of similars

The word 'homoeopathy' comes from the Greek, and may be translated as 'similar suffering'. In other words, the agent which can cause disease in a well person may be used to therapeutic advantage in the person who is sick and whose symptoms resemble those of the agent. This was a concept which had existed from the time of Hippocrates, but Samuel Hahnemann, the originator of homoeopathy as a modern medical theory, took the basic idea much further by developing it into a full therapeutic system. In doing so, he put forward a theory of health and disease which ran completely opposite to the current medical thinking of his own day and ours (this latter generally referred to as 'allopathy'). Instead of prescribing a drug which would oppose the symptoms of illness and suppress them, Hahnemann advocated the use of a medicinal

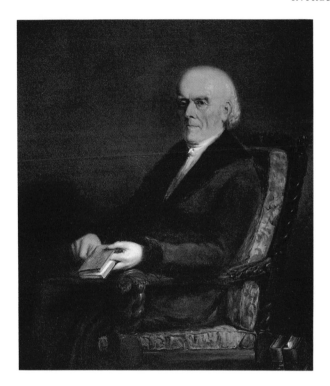

substance which worked with the body and encouraged it to throw off the symptoms by stimulating it to work more effectively.

Provings of remedies

In order to find out what effects a medicinal substance would have on an individual in good health, Hahnemann carried out a series of controlled experiments on himself and other volunteers. Those experiments he called 'provings'; they involve taking small amounts of a substance repeatedly and recording the effects. The people selected had to be in good health and ready to observe and record in meticulous detail any changes in their emotional or physical health during the period of the experiment. Today many hundreds of homoeopathic medicines are in use which have been proved in just this manner, and the process continues as new medicines are introduced.

The single dose

Because the provings were carried out using single substances rather than compounds of many ingredients, homoeopathic medicines are commonly given as single remedies in single doses. Reactions are then observed, and the decision is taken whether to wait longer, repeat, choose a stronger dose, or change the remedy altogether.

One of the main arguments in favour of the administration of single medicines is that it is very difficult to determine how effective a particular remedy has been if it is closely followed, or even mixed with another. Because of the method of proving single substances rather than mixtures, the information on medicinal effects is also not available for multiple compounds, so the effects of the interaction between these substances is something we cannot reliably be aware of.

The minimum dose

Parallel with the notion of treating by similars, Hahnemann also developed the theory that the dose of the medicine administered should be the smallest possible to effect a cure. This appears to have been a preoccupation of his from the time he spent in practice as an orthodox physician, during which he was increasingly appalled by the side effects he witnessed as a result of allopathic treatment. He, therefore, experimented using smaller and smaller doses of these similar medicinal substances, until he came to a point of dilution where orthodox science parted company with him. Although at this level of dilution, no molecules of the original substance could be found, Hahnemann discovered that these highly dilute medicines had a profound effect in

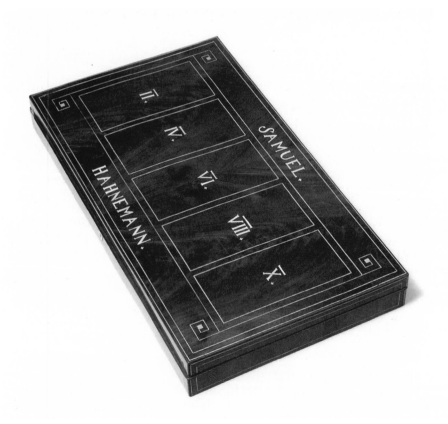

stimulating the process of healing in the body, provided they went through an additional process of vigorous shaking or 'sucussion' at each stage of dilution. In fact, he found that the higher the dilution and the further away he got from the material dose, the stronger the medicinal effect proved to be – as long as the similarity between the medicine and the patient's state still existed.

It must be emphasised that, for a substance to be homoeopathically active, the twin processes of dilution and sucussion must both be carried out; the dilution alone is not enough to render the remedy medicinally useful.

The importance of the individuality of the sick person

In homoeopathic practice each sick person is seen as an individual who will respond to ill health in his or her own particular way. A note is made of any changes from the patient's normal condition on the physical, mental, and emotional levels: it is the analysis of this vital information that will lead to the selection of the most appropriate homoeopathic medicine.

If we take an example of two people suffering from the common cold, we are likely to find that they share common symptoms of nasal discharge, sore throat, and a cough. This information in its general sense will do nothing to lead us to the appropriate homoeopathic medicine, because it conveys nothing of the way the individual is expressing his or her illness.

In order to discover this, we need to enquire far more deeply into the individual characteristics of the symptoms to establish a sharper picture. Upon closer questioning we may discover that one person complains of a scanty, clear, burning nasal discharge, while the other has a profuse, yellow-green, thick and bland secretion. The first person has been unbearably chilly since catching the cold, and feels happiest hugging the fire, while the other also feels chilly but is generally much worse for stuffy rooms and better for fresh air. Our chilly individual with the nasal discharge that burns the nostrils may also have noticed since the onset of the cold that she has felt unusually anxious, restless, and fussy, and has a cough that is very dry and troublesome at night. On the other hand, the sufferer with the aversion to stuffy rooms and the multicoloured mucus, may complain of feeling very weepy and in need of sympathy since the cold came on, and find that they have a very productive cough that is particularly loose in the mornings.

If we consider these two individuals in the light of the information given above, we see straight away how each one is expressing their symptoms of illness in their own individual way. Therefore, one would not give the same homoeopathic remedy to both, since their symptoms are not at all similar beyond the most general level, and it is the specifics that we are interested in. So we would suggest Arsenicum album in the first case, and Pulsatilla in the second. This is because the sick individual is being prescribed for, not the disease category in isolation.

How does homoeopathy differ from orthodox medicine?

In order to grasp fully the degree of contrast between the homoeopathic and orthodox medical approaches to ill health, it is necessary to consider the context within which Samuel Hahnemann developed his own ideas.

Origins

Samuel Hahnemann was born in 1755 in Meissen, Germany and qualified as a doctor in 1779. The more he observed of orthodox treatments in practice, the more alarmed he became at the appalling side effects that patients were suffering. It is easy to forget how barbaric things were in medical practice as recently as the late eighteenth century. Patients were commonly subjected to treatment involving toxic substances like Mercury in cases of venereal disease; bleeding practices were still much in vogue, including leeching, cupping, and venesection, and purging was often carried out to such a violent degree that patients were severely weakened.

By 1796, Hahnemann was so disturbed by what he had witnessed of current medical practice that he decided to refrain from practising as a physician and put his efforts instead into the translation of foreign medical texts. At the same time he conducted researches of his own into gentler ways of treating patients.

The major breakthrough came when he was translating Cullen's Materia Medica. Hahnemann was intrigued by Cullen's explanation for the effectiveness of Quinine in treating cases of malaria, but unsatisfied with his conclusion that it was the astringent properties of the substance that rendered it medicinally effective. Hahnemann decided that he would experiment by taking repeated doses of Quinine himself, and found that he began to develop symptoms of malaria which went away once he stopped taking the medicine. As a result of this experiment, he began the long and tortuous path of developing the theory and practice of homoeopathy: the treatment of sick individuals with similar substances rather than opposites. His clinical and theoretical work continued without interruption until his death in Paris in 1843.

After experimenting further along these lines with more medicinal substances, Hahnemann also began to work with more and more dilute forms of medicine in an effort to promote the gentlest and most effective form of treatment. At this point, he made a quantum leap in his thinking: to the process of dilution, he added the systematic repetition of sucussion or vigorous pounding. He found that both processes had to be carried out in order for a homoeopathically prepared remedy to be medicinally effective. This process came to be called 'potentization'.

The more he worked with patients using potentized medicines, the more he found that his observations ran counter to anything that could be explained by the scientific theory of his day. From the reactions he observed, the more dilute and sucussed a substance became (even to the point where there was no molecule of the original substance left), the more potent the effect appeared to be on the sick person, always providing the 'similarity' of the patient picture matched that of the remedy prescribed.

Concepts of vital energy

As Hahnemann continued to refine his ideas, he came to the conclusion that there must be some basic intelligence which governed the workings of the human body in good health. When this intelligence or 'vital force' came into conflict with a stressful stimulus which proved too strong for it to resist, symptoms of illness would be manifested in the person. These symptoms would be evidence of the body's own incomplete attempt to heal itself, thus providing clues as to the nature of the disturbance and essential information for the selection of the appropriate homoeopathic medicine.

Looked at in this way, symptoms of illness acquire a more benign identity than they do from the perspective of orthodox medicine.

The orthodox medical approach

Because modern medicine sees the human body as an object constantly under siege from hostile bacteria and viruses, many drug therapies work along the lines of searching for the 'magic bullet' which will kill off the offending microbe. Unlike homoeopathy, which attempts to stimulate and assist the body's own defence mechanism to overcome an infection, orthodox medicine works by identifying the individual organism, in order to eliminate it by administering the appropriate drug.

The nature of the drugs used are also quite different in orthodox practice when compared to homoeopathic selection of medicines. As we have previously pointed out, homoeopathic remedies are selected because their effect on the human economy is similar to the body's own self-defence mechanism. They thus enable the body to fight the disease stimulus more effectively. Allopathic or orthodox drugs, however, work on a totally different basis, since they are chosen on the basis of their countering the disease by producing an opposite effect. Everyday examples of these would include antacids to dilute over-acidity in the stomach, laxatives to deal with constipation, and anti-inflammatories to dampen down inflammation. Because such drugs work by countering symptoms, patients often have to continue taking them on a long-term basis to keep the symptoms under control. The homoeopathic approach is centred on helping the body to work more efficiently so that it can throw off and overcome symptoms itself; consequently, the long-term aim of homoeopathic treatment is to get the body sufficiently in balance so that medicinal intervention is unnecessary unless and until the body is again overwhelmed by stress.

Common problems with the orthodox medical approach to health and disease

The importance of the whole person

Unfortunately, because orthodox medical diagnosis puts so much emphasis on the common symptoms of disease in its selection of the appropriate drug therapy, it is easy to lose sight of the individual person in the pursuit of diagnosis. As a result, people who are ill often feel that they have become primarily a walking case of whatever they are suffering from; a feeling which is often reinforced by the battery of investigative tests to which they may be subjected.

Because orthodox medicine seems to think of good health as the absence of disease rather than the positive acquiring of a healthy and well-regulated body, this has often led to people expecting a pill for every minor problem that arises. This is largely because doctors have lost sight of the human body as an entity that has a defence mechanism of its own, which, when healthy, can fight off transient illness itself. As a result, many people have lost touch with steps they can take to aid their body through short-term infections like the common cold. Sensible supportive measures of keeping fluid intake high, having a light and easily digested diet, avoiding extremes of heat and chill in the environment, and taking a few days rest are all likely to assist the body in its fight against infection. Unfortunately, many of us expect a magic pill to rid us of unpleasant symptoms, ignoring the messages our body is sending us that we may need to take it easy for a few days.

When homoeopathy is used effectively, it is unlikely to abort symptoms of the common cold in their tracks, but it will support the body through the various stages so that the infection will pass more quickly and cause a minimum amount of complications. Because homoeopathy is working to assist the body in its fight, any measures that can be taken to help the struggle will be supportive of homoeopathic treatment. This is why in this book you will find extended sections in each chapter on general measures that can be taken in addition to prescribing homoeopathic medicines.

Because homoeopathic medicines are selected on the basis of matching the individual's symptom picture with the appropriate homoeopathic remedy, any changes that have appeared in the individual since the onset of the illness will be worth noting. These changes are not restricted to any physical symptoms that have appeared, but also refer to any emotional changes which may have surfaced since the illness commenced. It is very noticeable that people may experience any of the following reactions as a result of feeling unwell: tearfulness, irritability, excitability, withdrawal,

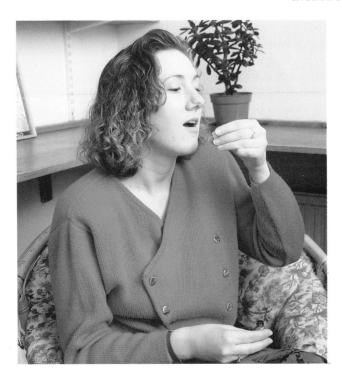

or anxiety. Any change on this emotional level is as relevant to the selection of the appropriate homoeopathic remedy as detailed information about aches and pains, nausea, mucus discharges, or fever.

There are some infections where orthodox medicine has little to offer in the way of drug therapy because the relevant agent has not been developed. Generally speaking, many viral infections are left to themselves because, with some exceptions, anti-viral agents are not in broad use like antibiotics. Because the homoeopathic approach is starting from a completely different premise of boosting the body's ability to overcome the infection, it is of little relevance whether the infection is of bacterial or viral origin. As a result, there are fewer limitations on the appropriate use of homoeopathy for infectious illnesses.

How holistic is homoeopathy?

The term 'holistic medicine' is one that many of us are very familiar with these days. Books have been devoted not only to the exploration of holistic therapies, but also to the wider concept of holistic living.

As concern with our external environment grows, and as that environment appears to be increasingly compromised by the excesses of living in a highly industrialised society, it is hardly surprising that many people are becoming concerned about how they set about achieving and protecting an optimum level of good health for themselves and their families. For such people, protecting the ecology of the individual body is becoming as pertinent an issue as protecting the rainforests, or defending the lives of whales.

Homoeopathy is a system of healing which fits very well within this context, because of its concern with achieving and maintaining the integrity of the health of the individual person. Because the medicines used do not have the unpleasant side effects of more toxic drugs, they provide a gentle but extremely effective way of stimulating the body back to good health. Of course, homoeopathy is not unique in occupying this position, since it has much in common with other therapies that one would broadly call holistic. These are therapies that also stress the need to get the individual person back to a state of good health rather than merely remove or suppress symptoms. They include acupuncture, herbalism, ayurvedic medicine, chiropractic and osteopathy.

Because homoeopathy is genuinely concerned with the impact of the environment on the physical, emotional, and mental levels of the individual, you will find that homoeopathic medicines are rarely selected on the basis of physical symptoms alone. There are, of course, some very straightforward first-aid situations where it would be needless to probe into the patient's state of emotional well-being. A sprained ankle or a bad bruise from a fall can be effectively prescribed for on the basis of detailed physical symptoms alone. Once one gets into the realm of stomach upsets, colds and 'flu, or transient anxiety states, however, any information about emotional changes may provide a vital clue to the selection of the appropriate remedy. If we go a step further and consider the homoeopathic practitioner taking the case of a chronically sick individual, the question of the patient's emotional environment becomes even more crucial to the enterprise.

Who can benefit from homoeopathy?

Generally speaking, homoeopathy is a system of medicine that is potentially helpful to anyone. Many homoeopaths say that there are no barriers to homoeopathy in treating diseases, but that there are some individuals who have more responsive defence mechanisms or immune systems than others.

Of course, there are serious diseases where the prognosis will be more disheartening than others, and there will always be stubborn cases where response is slow in forthcoming. If someone has suffered from an illness for many years and has undergone long courses of suppressive therapy, they are likely to find that they will take longer to respond than a young child who has recently fallen ill within the context of general good health.

Age is not a stumbling block to the suitability of homoeopathy as a therapy: babies can be treated as effectively as the elderly. Homoeopathy is also not limited to the treatment of humans: farm and domestic animals have been effectively helped by the use of veterinary homoeopathy.

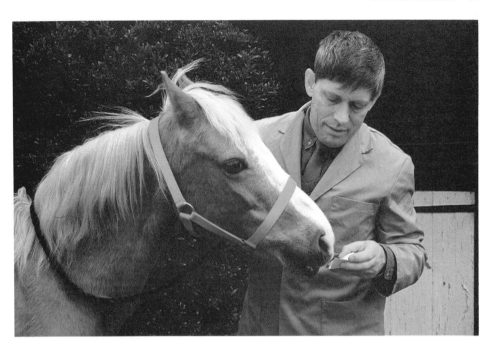

Homoeopathy in the United Kingdom

One may select a homoeopathic practitioner in this country from two possible avenues of training. There are orthodox doctors who have obtained an additional training in homoeopathy. These may work in the National Health Service, as homoeopathic consultants at one of the homoeopathic hospitals, or in private practice. Lists of addresses are given at the end of this book which will identify where the hospitals are, and where you may obtain a list of orthodox doctors who practice homoeopathy.

It is also possible to consult a homoeopathic practitioner who has not received a formal orthodox medical training, but has a thorough grounding in homoeopathy. These practitioners currently tend to work privately outside the National Health Service. For an up-to-date register of professional homoeopaths who have undergone a minimum of four years' training, contact the Society of Homoeopaths.

You will find that homoeopathic medicines are increasingly available from high street chemists and health food shops. There are also pharmacies which specialise in the preparation and retailing of homoeopathic medicines. These will usually supply remedies by post if you order by letter or by telephone. (Addresses and telephone numbers for all of the above will be found in the Useful Addresses section at the back of the book.)

Homoeopathy abroad

Homoeopathy flourishes in India today where it has received official recognition as a separate medical system, with a government-approved Central Homoeopathic Council. Homoeopathic treatment is available widely from 200,000 or more practitioners, of whom 70,000 are registered with state boards. India has the largest number of homoeopathic hospitals, and training may be obtained from over 100 colleges.

In France, one may obtain homoeopathic remedies and treatment very easily from orthodox physicians who have taken additional training in homoeopathy. It was estimated in a recent survey that approximately 25 per cent of the French public have used homoeopathic medicine, and that 11,000 doctors adopt it as a therapy. Unfortunately, remedies may only be prescribed in comparatively low doses (nothing above 30c) which tends to limit clinical flexibility. Although homoeopathic remedies are freely available in over 20,000 pharmacies, emphasis is often put on the use of complex or compound preparations of remedies which may be used more routinely than a more holistic practitioner would recommend.

Combination remedies may also be found in Germany, where homoeopathy also enjoys a high profile among medical practitioners. Other countries where homoeopathy is well established or gaining in popularity include Mexico, Argentina, Brazil, Australia, South Africa, New Zealand, Holland and Greece. In the United States, where homoeopathy was a strong rival of orthodox medicine until the early years of this century, the system went into severe decline for several decades, but over the past 10 years a revival has taken place in a number of states. Homoeopathy has also started to develop in Russia and Eastern Europe.

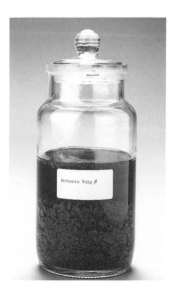

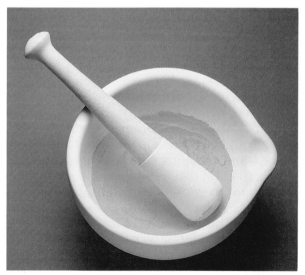

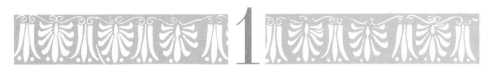

1

PRACTICAL HOMOEOPATHY

What conditions are appropriate for self-help?

You will find that certain health problems are conspicuous by their absence from this book. If you want to find out how to self-prescribe for eczema, migraines, asthma, or period problems, I'm afraid you will not find them listed in the self-help sections. The reason for this is quite simple, and lies in the contrast between acute and chronic forms of disease. It is *not* because homoeopathy can't help.

If a problem is classed as **acute**, this does not refer to the severity of the condition. It is a term which defines a self-limiting condition, in other words, one that will clear up of its own accord given the right conditions and enough time for the body to deal with it. Good examples of acute problems include colds, 'flu, food poisoning, and childhood infectious illnesses. You will find that the conditions covered by this book generally fall into the acute category.

Chronic problems, unlike acutes, are much less likely to resolve themselves, no matter how much time and ample opportunity the body is given to recuperate. The general pattern of chronic illness is that of repeated flare-ups which may go into remission for a time, but will always tend to return. Good examples of chronic problems would include asthma, hay fever, eczema, psoriasis, and irritable bowel syndrome. It is true to say that some chronic conditions will give rise to acute exacerbations within the chronic condition, but these should not be confused with an acute problem which arises without the bedrock of a chronic problem.

Generally speaking, acute conditions respond well to self-help prescribing, but chronic problems need help from a qualified practitioner. Case management of chronic conditions can be complicated, and the training of a professional is required to steer the patient towards a state of improved health. This is especially true of the management of skin conditions, since homoeopaths generally view a persistent skin eruption as indicative of a deeper, underlying, inherited disorder which needs to be dealt with before the whole person can enjoy improved health. If the skin condition is combined with the patient suffering from a more internal disorder such as asthma, very careful case management is needed to deal with the overall improvement of the case. In cases such as these, the practitioner needs to be prepared for any complications which may arise during treatment, and must constantly use his or her professional judgement to assess how the patient is progressing.

You will find that hay fever is the one chronic condition that has been included in this book. The reasoning behind this is simple: for many people, the symptoms of hay fever during the summer closely resemble those of the common cold. In this situation, finding a helpful homoeopathic remedy can be as straightforward as selecting the most appropriate remedy for an acute bout of cold. You will notice, however, that a statement appears at the top of the hay fever table advising anyone suffering from it to seek professional help. This is because acute prescribing will do nothing to alleviate the underlying problem, and relief will only be obtained on a short-term basis. If professional help is sought for the condition, results on a long-term basis are likely to be much more satisfactory.

The omission of any other conditions which may be defined as acutes will have been done on the basis of personal judgement. Headaches, for example, do not appear, since it has been my experience that it can be very difficult for the beginner to differentiate between various sorts of head pain. In the situation where individualising characteristics can be hard to isolate, results can be disappointing. This is a purely subjective opinion, and does not mean that you will find headaches omitted from other homoeopathic self-help manuals.

You will also find that there is a strong emphasis in each section on which symptoms indicate that you may be getting out of your depth and that you need a professional opinion. Never be hesitant about getting help if you suspect a condition could be serious: in this situation it is always most prudent to err on the cautious side.

How do I learn more about homoeopathic self-help?

I would strongly urge anyone who has bought this book to attend one of the many classes in homoeopathic first-aid or self-help that are held across the country. It has been my own experience that a book can teach one a great deal about the basics of self-prescribing, but inevitably there will always be questions in the reader's mind which may not be covered by the information in the book. Once you have become familiar with this book, attending a homoeopathic self-help class will give you the opportunity to discuss issues with other beginners like yourself, and your questions can be answered by the practitioner who is running the class.

If you would like to obtain information about self-help classes in your area I would suggest you contact your local library, education authority (extra-mural studies), local Homoeopathic Group, or Homoeopathic College.

Where can I obtain homoeopathic medicines?

You will find that there are increasing numbers of outlets for the sale of homoeopathic medicines as the demand for homoeopathic treatment is growing. Many high street chemists now have stocks of basic homoeopathic medicines, and health food shops usually provide a similar choice.

There are pharmacies which also manufacture and supply homoeopathic medicines who are happy to deal with telephone orders. If you require any medicines which are less easily available, you will need to order from this source. Names and addresses of homoeopathic pharmacies are given in the Useful Addresses section at the end of this book.

You will find that you can obtain homoeopathic medicines in the form of large or small tablets, granules, pilules, powders or in liquid form as tinctures. Creams, ointments, lotions and tinctures are also available for external use.

Potencies

Most of the homoeopathic medicines that can be bought over the counter come in either 6c or 30c potency. The 'c' refers to the method of dilution that has been employed (in this case the centesimal scale of dilution). You may also come across remedies that have a 'd' or 'x' after the number, this refers to the decimal scale. In the centesimal form of dilution, the original substance to be rendered homoeopathically active is diluted in alcohol. One drop of this dilution is taken and added to 99 drops of distilled water or alcohol and vigorously shaken to give the first potency.

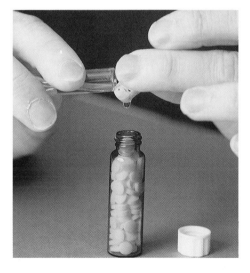
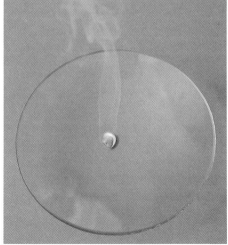

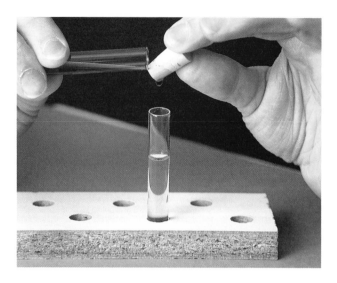

This process is repeated at each stage, taking one drop of the previous potency and adding it to 99 drops of dilutant. The same process is used for the decimal scale, but the proportion used is one drop of tincture to nine drops of alcohol or distilled water.

How to use this book

How do I decide which remedy to choose?

In order to use this book effectively to find the most appropriate homoeopathic medicine, you will need to do the following.

1 Using a notebook and pencil, write down any symptoms you have noticed since the onset of illness. These may refer to subjective changes as well as observable symptoms such as paleness in a person who normally has a healthy complexion.

2 Do remember that you are only interested in any changes from the normal state of the sick person. In other words, if someone is normally chilly, you would not attribute any importance to this. If, however, this person complained of feeling flushed and hot since their illness, this would be a valid symptom, because it signifies a change from the normal state for that individual.

3 Once you have listed all the symptoms you regard as being important, isolate any that you would regard as being peculiar. For instance, fever without thirst, chilliness with aversion to heat, or nausea that is better for eating. These are important symptoms as they may clinch your choice of remedy.

4 Try to identify a characteristic, or theme, running through the symptoms. You may find dryness a

major characteristic running through skin texture, sensations in the throat, and bowel movements. When you have a major thread like this running through the symptoms you have a head start.

5 Enquire if there has been a precipitating factor before illness set in such as exposure to cold winds, or several nights' disturbed sleep, or a severe fright or shock. This is always worth noting.

6 Establish what makes the patient feel generally better or worse. This can apply to things which relieve or aggravate specific symptoms, or which have a general systemic effect on the patient.

7 Always note any changes on the emotional level which have occurred since the illness set in. Weepiness in a normally cheerful individual, or anxiety and restlessness in a normally relaxed person, are always symptoms of value.

8 By now you should have a fairly long list of symptoms which you can divide by putting under headings of **causitive factors**, **general symptoms**, and **modalities** (things which make the patient generally feel better or worse).

9 Do remember that the general symptom heading can have a very wide scope, referring to any changes from normal on both physical and emotional levels.

10 Now turn to the appropriate table in the relevant section of the book. Look down the left hand column entitled **Type** to see which category is likely to fit most closely to the group of symptoms you have

on paper. If there is a causitive factor, this will help you a great deal at this stage. This column will also give you information about what stage of illness you may be thinking of, in other words, whether one is thinking about early onset of a more established stage.

11 If you have found the category you want, check the information given under the next column entitled **General indications** and see how it corresponds to the general symptoms you have noted. It is unlikely that you will ever find a perfect match between the two, so don't worry if you can't find all the symptoms you have noted under that heading. What you will need to assess is whether the most important elements of the general indications cover the symptoms you have seen as important. To give an example: one would not consider Belladonna for someone with a cold unless they were very hot, dry, and feverish, and the cold had developed quite suddenly. If someone had a cold which had taken a long time to develop, looked pale, sweaty, and withdrawn, and felt very chilly, then clearly Belladonna will not fit and one would look elsewhere for the appropriate remedy.

12 If you are unsure what symptoms represent the key features of a homoeopathic remedy, turn to the section at the back of the book entitled **Keynotes**. This will give you a quick overview of the essential features running through each remedy.

13 If you feel satisfied that the match between the symptoms of your patient and the homoeopathic remedy you are considering are close enough, look at the columns entitled **Worse from** and **Better for**. If you feel that these also apply in general to the sick person, then it looks like you have found the most appropriate remedy.

14 Remember, what you are looking for is the information which characterises what is individual in the sick person's symptoms. Always try to find out what it is that makes the person's case of 'flu or food poisoning different from another's. Common symptoms such as vomiting, sore throat, or cough will not help you at all in your search for the appropriate homoeopathic remedy. You must always try to define how these broad symptoms affect the individual in the way they perceive pain, the colour and texture of their discharges, and how these specific symptoms affect their systems as a whole.

15 You will soon observe that the same medicines appear under different sections. For instance, Pulsatilla appears in the tables for Indigestion, Coughs, Colds, and Chicken Pox, while Arsenicum Album will appear in tables for Vomiting, Anxiety, Coughs, and Influenza. By using these tables and the Keynotes at the back of the book, you will begin to grasp the concept of these being multi-faceted medicines that cover a range of complaints in their own individual way. As you become more familiar with their use you will begin to appreciate how each remedy has individual characteristics of its own, just as the sick person manifests his or her own disease in a way that is particular to them.

How to take homoeopathic medicines

Homoeopathic medicines are normally in tablet form, but topical treatments such as tinctures and creams are also available for wounds or burns.

1 Tip out a single dose of your selected remedy (a single dose being one tablet) onto a clean spoon.

2 Do not wash the tablets down with water, but suck them as you would a sweet in a clean mouth. Bear in mind that a clean mouth does not involve cleaning your teeth before taking the remedy, but refers more to the necessity of avoiding eating, drinking or cleaning your teeth too close to taking your remedy. It's a good idea to try to leave half an hour either side of eating or drinking.

3 Some homoeopaths strongly recommend that you avoid the use of tea, coffee, peppermint, or the application of strong-smelling rubs involving camphor. These are some of the substances that are thought to interfere with the effective action of homoeopathic medicines. I would suggest that it is a good idea to avoid these if you are beginning to use homoeopathy, since it avoids an element of potential confusion if it looks like the remedy you have selected is not working.

4 Store remedies away from strong light, odours, or extreme variations of temperature. A fairly cool, dark place is usually most suitable. If your remedies are kept under these conditions they will remain active, since they do not have a short 'shelf life'.

5 If you accidentally spill some tablets out of the bottle, do not put them back in, throw them away.

6 If you are giving the remedy to a small child who has difficulty sucking a tablet, you can crush the tablet between two clean spoons and put the powder under the tongue to be absorbed, or rub it along the gums.

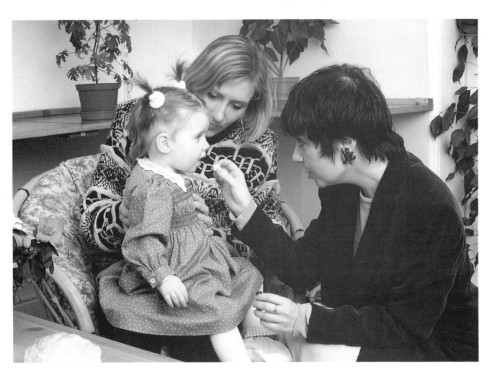

How often to repeat the remedy

1 Take your first dose of the indicated remedy (a single dose being one tablet). Wait for half an hour; if there is no change, repeat the remedy. You can repeat the dose for up to three doses at half-hourly intervals.

2 If you notice an improvement by the second or third dose, **stop** taking the remedy. This is an indication your body is now doing the work for itself, and that continuing the remedy will not be necessary unless the symptoms recur. Once again, as soon as you notice an improvement, stop taking the remedy.

3 The repetition suggested above is the recommended dose for a condition of sudden and recent onset, as in the case of food poisoning. If, however, your condition has been building up over a few days and appears to be more stubborn, you are likely to respond more favourably to repetition of the appropriate remedy three or four times daily over a period of three to four days. As before, once improvement takes place, **stop** taking the remedy.

4 If there is no improvement after waiting the suggested time, take another look at the appropriate table and see if another remedy may be more suitable. If one remedy hasn't worked, there is no problem of incompatibility of medicines in moving on to another which may be more effective. Because the remedies work at a sub-molecular level, there is no risk of any chemical residue being left in the tissues which might spark off a toxic reaction.

5 You will find that most health food shops and pharmacies now stock homoeopathic medicines in either 6c or 30c strength. I would suggest that if the condition is fairly mild and of recent onset you try the indicated remedy for you in 6c potency, and move on to the 30c if you feel only marginal improvement with the lower dose. It would be appropriate to begin with a 12c (available from homoeopathic pharmacies) or 30c potency if the condition has been of longer duration and the symptoms are more severe.

6 Homoeopathic medicines are not designed to be taken on a long-term basis for acute (short-lived) disorders. If you feel that you need to take them on a daily basis to achieve the desired effect, the chances are that you need more long-term, 'constitutional' treatment from a homoeopathic practitioner.

7 Above all, if you are at all confused and feeling a bit lost, always **seek professional help**.

Do remember that it is the potency and frequency of repetition of the remedy that determines the strength and length of action of the remedy, rather than the size of the dose. In other words, if one gives one, two, or five tablets at the same time it still counts as a single dose of the remedy. If, however, one gave a single tablet to the patient every ten minutes for an hour, this would count as six doses, since the remedy is being administered repeatedly.

Which remedies should I buy?

I'm afraid it is very difficult to be absolutely specific about the exact number of remedies needed in the average basic first-aid kit, since one person's needs will not be the same as another's. For instance, anyone with babies and young children in their family is likely to need a kit which features remedies such as Chamomilla and Colocynthis that are especially useful for childhood problems. These are not so likely to be indicated or useful in the kit required by people without children.

However, I would suggest that the following list of remedies would provide a good starter kit for someone who needs to have a basic range of the most frequently indicated homoeopathic medicines.

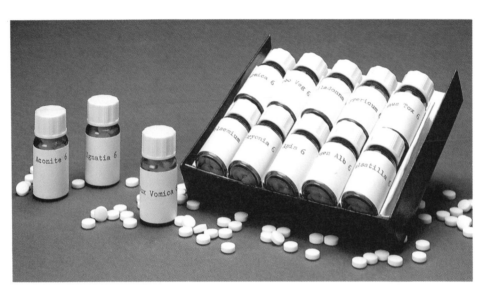

Aconite	*Carbo veg*	*Nux vomica*
Arnica	*Gelsemium*	*Phosphorus*
Arsenicum album	*Hypericum*	*Pulsatilla*
Belladonna	*Ignatia*	*Rhus tox*
Bryonia		

Once you have this basic range of remedies, I would suggest useful additions would include the following:

Apis	*Ipecac*	*Lachesis*
Chamomilla	*Ledum*	*Ruta*
Ferrum phos	*Lycopodium*	*Staphysagria*
Hepar sulph	*Mercurius*	*Veratrum album*

In addition, I would also suggest you obtain the following creams and tinctures for topical administration:

Hypercal tincture (T.M.) – to be used diluted on cuts and grazes.
Calendula cream – to be applied after Hypercal tincture on cuts and grazes to ensure the wound remains free of infection, and to help speed healing of tissue.
Urtica urens tincture – to be diluted and applied to minor burns and scalds.

These are, of course, arbitrary lists and should in no way be considered exhaustive. There are many more 'basic' homoeopathic remedies, all of them useful, but the above should provide the beginner with a basis on which to build.

What potency should I buy?

Once again, this is a rather difficult question to answer, since different situations often require different potencies of the appropriate homoeopathic remedy. For an explanation of potencies and their range please see the section entitled Potencies on page 21. I would suggest that you initially buy your remedies in 6c potency, and supplement these with the same remedies in 12c and 30c later. Do not worry unduly about selecting the optimum potency in the early days: if you have selected the most appropriate homoeopathic remedy, use either a 6c, 12c, or 30c, remembering that the 6c potency will require more frequent repetition than the higher potencies.

When prescribing for children the same basic principles apply as for adults. You should bear in mind that conditions often develop more quickly and violently in children than in adults, and the chosen homoeopathic remedy may need to be repeated frequently in order to maintain an improvement. If the selected remedy in a 6c potency seems to be only giving partial or short-lived relief, consider moving on to the same remedy in a 30c potency. As always, do not repeat the remedy while an improvement is holding, only if there are signs that the symptoms are returning. If you are at all concerned about the seriousness of your child's condition, always get professional advice.

HOMOEOPATHIC FIRST-AID

Accidents and injuries

Most advice given to people who have sustained a non-life-threatening injury tends to be limited to suggestions about rest, judicious use of painkillers, and the employment of supports (such as putting a limb in plaster while healing is taking place). There is a basic acknowledgement that, given the best conditions, the body will heal traumatised tissue itself, and that this takes time. Clearly, more life-threatening injuries or accidents will call for more radical measures such as emergency surgery and drugs; but even in this situation, once the emergency phase is over, time is once again acknowledged as the prime healing agent.

Homoeopathic medicines and accidents and injuries

Prescribing for accidents and injuries is one of the many areas where homoeopathic medicine comes into its own. Use of Arnica in an injury not only helps deal with the initial shock but also limits bruising by promoting the re-absorption of blood while minimising pain. Symphytum promotes the knitting of bones in a fracture and eases pain, while Calendula acts as a natural antiseptic, slowing down bleeding and aiding the healing of tissue. In all of these situations, the homoeopathic medicines are acting as catalysts, speeding up the processes which would naturally happen in the body, given time. The advantages of judicious homoeopathic prescribing are obvious in a situation where time is acknowledged as the best healer.

How to select the appropriate homoeopathic medicine

You will find homoeopathic prescribing for accidents and injuries a little different to the prescribing outlined in other sections of this book. This is because, for many conditions in this section, initial prescribing is much more routinist than in other conditions such as indigestion or coughs and colds. For instance, you will quickly notice that Arnica is universally recommended as the first remedy to take internally if there has been any shock or trauma to the system following injury. In other situations where more differentiation is required – as in **Sprains and Strains** – follow the advice given below.

1 Turn to the table entitled **Sprains and Strains**. Let us say that

Arnica has helped the acute phase of injury enormously, but you are left with residual pain that is not being resolved by the remedy. Look down the left hand column entitled **Type** to identify which category your symptoms fall into. If you are in pain once you begin movement, but feel much better once you have got going, the chances are that the column entitled 'Sprains and strains that feel better for continued movement' is the one for you.

2 Check with the **General indications** that these symptoms fit with your own. If you have pains associated with muscular over-exertion that feel relieved by continued, gentle movement, then it looks as though you are on the right track.

3 Finally, check the **Worse from** and **Better for** columns to see if these also fit. Do bear in mind that these two columns do not just refer to what makes your sprain or strain better or worse, but also to what might make you *generally* feel better or worse. So, if you have definitely noticed that you feel worse for exposure to damp and cold, but taking a warm bath or staying warm in bed helps your pain, the chances are that Rhus tox is the remedy for you.

For information on how to take the appropriate remedy, see the section entitled **How to take homoeopathic medicines** in the chapter on **Practical Homoeopathy**; exactly the same principles apply.

Remember that in first-aid situations it is appropriate to take one remedy internally, and to use another topically on the skin in cream or lotion form. For example, if you have sustained a cut after a fall, it is fine to take Arnica internally while you bathe the cut with diluted Calendula tincture. Do bear in mind that Arnica cream should only be applied to bruises where the skin is unbroken; *do not* apply it to cuts or grazes. In the latter situation, Calendula would be the most appropriate choice of ointment or cream.

Cuts and bruises

Type	General indications	Worse from	Better for	Remedy name
Simple cuts and grazes	Cuts which are straightforward with no signs of sepsis. The remedy may be taken in cream, or diluted tincture which may be applied directly to the wound	Chill	Being still	Calendula

Type	General indications	Worse from	Better for	Remedy name
Deep cuts with nerve involvement	Very useful for injuries to parts rich in nerves: fingers, toes and soles of feet. Pains are shooting, and there is a general hypersensitivity to touch	Touch. Moving	Being still	Hypericum
Incised wounds	Clean cuts with stinging, lacerated sensations. Often indicated in injury from sharp instruments	Motion. Pressure	Heat	Staphysagria
Simple bruising, early stages	Sore, aching and bruised sensations which make someone feel very restless and uncomfortable. Also indicated for the general systemic trauma following a fall or accident. The remedy may be taken internally, or applied to the bruised area in cream form, **provided the surface of the skin has not been cut**	Exertion. Touch	Resting with head lower than the body	Arnica
Black eyes or bruises that feel better from cold applications	May be indicated after the Arnica has reached the end of its usefulness. Often helps ease the pain and speed up the healing of bruised tissue around the eye area	Heat. Moving	Cool air. Cold bathing. Resting	Ledum
Bruising as a result of injury to the eyeball or bones around the eye	May be indicated after Arnica if swelling has subsided, but pain persists. Often helpful after injury to the eye from a blunt object	Touch		Symphytum
Bruises of the shin-bone, knee-cap or elbow	Very strongly indicated for bruises involving the periosteum (the membranous sheath that provides a covering for bones). Sensations are generally sore, bruised and lame	Lying. Sitting. Going up or down stairs	Warmth. Rubbing	Ruta

Type	General indications	Worse from	Better for	Remedy name
Very deep bruising to tissues	May be indicated after a heavy blow which results in bruising of deep tissue, e.g. a blow to the breasts. May also be of use after bruising of deeper tissue following surgery	Touch. Hot bath	Moving. Cold applied locally	Bellis perennis

The following will be helpful in addition to selecting the appropriate homoeopathic remedy:

1 Where the skin has been broken, be sure to bathe the wound, removing any dirt which is visible. Examine the wound thoroughly before applying a sterile dressing to check no dirt has been left embedded in the skin.

2 When bathing a cut, diluted Calendula or 'Hypercal' tincture in boiled, cooled water makes an excellent antiseptic solution. Calendula will help speed up healing of lacerated tissue, aid in stopping bleeding, and act as a natural antiseptic inhibiting infection. When diluting the tincture use one part of tincture to 10 parts of cooled, boiled water.

3 Calendula cream also makes an excellent antiseptic agent when applied to clear skin after bathing with diluted Calendula tincture. For grazed wounds Calendula ointment is more appropriate.

4 Bear in mind that a wide cut may need stitches. If not, bringing the edges of the wound together and covering the area with a sterile gauze bandage may be sufficient.

5 If bruising has occurred and the skin has not been broken, applying ice-packs to the injured area for 20 or 30 minutes will help reduce swelling.

6 For bruised tissue where the skin has not been broken, Arnica cream may be applied directly to the skin. This will act in tandem with internal administration of the remedy, relieving pain and speeding up the healing process.

If any of the following occur, professional help is likely to be needed:

1 Any bleeding which is profuse or associated with numbness or tingling associated with loss of strength.

2 Deep cuts sustained to the chest, face, or abdomen.

3 Deep, wide cuts which refuse to be held together with adhesive bandages. In cases like these, stitches are likely to be required.

4 If dirt is very deeply embedded and cannot be expelled by bathing and cleaning.

5 Any sign of infection around a wound, especially affecting the

palm of the hand or the underside of the fingers.

6 If someone shows signs of repeated easy bruising.

Puncture wounds

Type	General indications	Worse from	Better for	Remedy name
Puncture wounds feel better for cold applications	Redness and swelling with throbbing pains. The wound feels cold to the touch, and feels better for bathing the affected part with cold water. Stinging and pricking pains. The first remedy to consider in puncture wounds	Warmth	Cold bathing	Ledum
Puncture wounds with lots of pink, swollen skin	Lots of sensations of heat and stinging pains that feel much worse for warmth. The site of the wound is extremely swollen and puffy	Heat. Touch	Cool air. Cold bathing	Apis
Puncture wounds with sharp, shooting pains	Intolerable shooting pains with lacerating sensations. Pains shoot from the site of injury along the affected limb. Wound feels extremely sensitive to touch	Touch. Jarring		Hypericum

The following measures will be helpful in addition to selecting the appropriate homoeopathic remedy:

1 Try to clean the wound as thoroughly as you can, letting it bleed for a while to remove foreign bodies, germs and debris. If bleeding is severe, apply pressure to the appropriate point above the artery, but do not exert pressure over the wound itself. This helps to avoid pushing any foreign bodies deeper into the wound.

2 Soaking the wounded area is helpful since it has the dual advantage of keeping the wound open to expel any foreign bodies and germs, while it also brings blood to the area which will speed the healing process. This may be done up to four times a day for about 20 minutes, for as long as the pain continues.

3 Applying diluted 'Hypercal' tincture to the wound will greatly ease the pain and speed up healing while the appropriate homoeopathic remedy is being taken internally.

If any of the following occur professional help is likely to be needed:

1 Puncture wounds that remain tender in excess of two days.

2 Puncture wounds affecting the hands rather than the fingers.

3 Any sign of infection around a puncture wound.

4 Deep puncture wounds or those that are located anywhere except the extremities.

5 Joints affected by puncture wounds, especially if you observe any signs of infection.

6 If you suspect the onset of tetanus, it is advisable to seek professional help.

Strains and sprains

Type	General indications	Worse from	Better for	Remedy name
Early stage with much swelling and bruised pain	Lots of swelling around the affected area with signs of inflammation and bruising. Pains are sore and aching and feel worse for movement. Also useful for general shock associated with injury. May be useful for general strain associated with overexertion	Moving. Touch		Arnica
Strains and sprains which are much worse for the slightest movement	Lots of inflammation with rosy red swelling, but not as extreme as sprains and strains requiring Arnica. Generally much better for keeping still and very much worse for moving. Pains feel stitching	Slight moving. Continued motion	Rest. Pressure	Bryonia
Sprains and strains that feel better for continued movement	Often needed like Bryonia once the most acute stage of injury has passed. Symptoms are often connected to muscular over-exertion. May feel pain once movement has begun, but begin to feel relief once movement is underway	Initial motion. At night. Exposure to cold and damp	Continued motion. Warmth. Warm bathing	Rhus tox

Type	General indications	Worse from	Better for	Remedy name
Torn ligaments and tendons: later stages	Particular affinity for ankle and wrist joints. Pains may feel bruised and aching and may have been helped initially by Arnica and Rhus tox. May respond badly to cold. Especially useful for frozen shoulder and tennis elbow	Cold. Resting. Walking out of doors	Warm. Moving indoors	Ruta
Sprained ankles which feel better for cold	Injured part may feel cold to the touch, and the pain may be relieved by cold applications or cold bathing. Lots of stiffness with pain	Heat. Walking. At night	Cool bathing. Resting	Ledum

Apart from selecting the appropriate homoeopathic remedy, the following measures will be helpful in speeding up the healing process:

1 Apply ice-packs to the injured area if there is heat and swelling and elevate the affected limb.

2 Warm applications may be soothing after the first 24 to 48 hours. Hot or warm bathing may also be soothing.

3 Rest the injured part as much as possible, since over-use of an injured tendon or ligament may cause further damage.

4 If injury to the joint is mild, gentle massage may be very soothing.

5 Do not be tempted to start over-using the joint before it has fully healed. Tendons and ligaments may take anything from six weeks to heal.

If any of the following occur, professional help is strongly advised:

1 If the joint cannot be straightened.

2 Any visible signs of distortion or looseness of the joint.

3 Marked swelling or pain which does not subside after a reasonable time.

4 If there are any signs of the limb beyond the injury looking blue, or feeling cold or numb.

5 If a joint cannot bear weight or be used for between 12 and 24 hours after the injury has occurred.

6 Take especial care with children who fall on an outstretched hand and injure their wrist. Fractures of the bones of the wrist often occur this way and special care may be needed in picking them up.

Fractures

Type	General indications	Worse from	Better for	Remedy name
Immediately after the injury	General indications of systemic shock, trauma, and local tenderness. The person may feel dazed after the injury, and there is likely to be a lot of localised bruising and swelling	Being touched	Lying with head low	Arnica
Severe pain associated in fractures with little swelling	Pains are violent and aching and may be associated with feelings of systemic weakness	Pressure to injured part. Cold	Being spoken to	Eupatorium perfoliatum
Fractured ribs which feel much worse from the slightest movement	Because of the sensitivity of movement, the injured person feels they must keep very still. Longs to take a deep breath in, but can't because of the pain. May get relief from lying on the injured side	Moving. Heat	Lying motionless. Firm pressure to area	Bryonia
Fractures which have been set in place	Useful for the stage when the initial swelling and pain have subsided, and the knitting of the bone needs to be speeded up. Since this remedy is very efficient at promoting the speedy knitting of bone, always make sure the bones have been set in alignment before administering it	Touch		Symphytum
Fractures which refuse to knit speedily, even after the use of Symphytum	Slow-knitting bones with sensations of numbness and stiffness as well as pain	Change of weather. Cold	Warm, dry weather	Calc phos

In addition to selecting the appropriate homoeopathic medicine, the following measures will be helpful:

1 If you suspect an injury may involve a fracture, keep the limb as still as possible and seek professional help.

2 If the skin has not been broken, ice-packs will be useful as a way of keeping swelling down.

If any of the following occur, professional help is indicated:

1 If the person who has sustained the injury seems faint, sweaty or pale.

2 If you suspect a serious injury of the neck or back, or if the person is unconscious.

3 Any signs of distortion to the injured area.

4 Indications of blueness, coldness or numbness associated with the limb beyond the injured area.

5 Any possible fracture to the thigh or pelvis.

6 Signs of severe bruising or bleeding under the skin around the injured area.

7 If the limb is unusable within 12 hours of the injury.

Burns

Type	General indications	Worse from	Better for	Remedy name
First degree burns	Stinging pains with intense burning	Touch		Urtica urens. May be used internally, or as a **diluted** tincture directly on the skin. Also consider Calendula tincture
Second degree burns	Stinging pains with intense burning			Use Hypericum tincture diluted and Urtica urens internally. Once blisters have broken, switch to diluted Calendula tincture

Type	General indications	Worse from	Better for	Remedy name
Third degree burns (1)	Cutting, burning and smarting pains – skin feels raw. Pain and inflammation are violently acute. Acute blistering	Warmth	Cold applied locally	Cantharis internally
Third degree burns (2)	Tearing, drawing, burning pains leading to trembling. Indicated for the effects of deep burns. May also be helpful in resolving old burns that have not been resolved	Draught	Even temperature	Causticum
Electrical burns				Phosphorus

In addition to giving the appropriate homoeopathic remedy, it is worthwhile bearing the following in mind:

1 Treating first and straightforward second degree burns may be carried out at home. Third degree burns and more serious second degree burns will need attention in hospital as soon as possible.

2 Avoid breaking blisters as this may lead to an infected wound. If a blister breaks spontaneously, use Calendula lotion, or diluted Calendula tincture to inhibit infection. Dressings should be changed two or three times a day.

3 For straightforward first degree burns, apply cold water to the burn until the pain has eased. Then apply the appropriate diluted tincture as well as taking the indicated remedy internally.

4 Do not try to remove any clothing from a third degree burn. While waiting for help try to reassure the injured person as much as possible.

If any of the following situations occur, you will need professional help:

1 Any third degree burn. Watch for symptoms of shock. These are confusion or unconsciousness; weakness; irregular or shallow breathing; coldness and pale skin.

2 Any sign of infection involving swelling, redness, or pus around the area of the burn.

Shock

Type	General indications	Worse from	Better for	Remedy name
Shock associated with physical trauma	Most often indicated after a fall or accident involving lots of bruising. Swelling, bruised pain, and the possible injuries to the head and neck would suggest the appropriateness of this remedy	Being approached. Touch	Lying with head low	Arnica
Shock symptoms with marked need for fresh air	State of collapse with skin which has a blue tinge and which feels cold and clammy to the touch. A strong desire may be expressed for being fanned, which alleviates the general condition	Warmth. Pressure of clothes	Being fanned. Cool air. Elevating feet	Carbo veg
Shock with severe anxiety and restlessness	Shock may follow a life-threatening situation, where the person may be left with a conviction that they are about to die. Breathing is rapid, and palpitations occur with a heightened anxiety state. Sweating may occur with marked trembling	Being chilled. Noise. Light	Rest. Open air	Aconite

While waiting for professional help, the following measures will be helpful in addition to giving the appropriate homoeopathic remedy:

1 Reassure the patient as much as possible.

2 Loosen clothing at the neck, waist and chest.

3 Try to avoid the patient being exposed to extremes of heat and cold.

4 On no account move the patient if you suspect a serious injury.

5 Legs may be elevated slightly higher than the chest.

6 Get help as quickly as possible.

Heat/sunstroke

Type	General indications	Worse from	Better for	Remedy name
Sunstroke with throbbing headache made better by bending the head backwards	Bright red, dry skin which radiates heat. Hot sensations may alternate with chills, and there may be an absence of thirst with fever. Throbbing sensations with headache are likely to be aggravated by lying down in a darkened room. Pains move in a downward direction	Noise. Light. Jarring. Lying flat	Bending head back. Dark rooms	Belladonna
Sunstroke with throbbing headaches made worse by bending head back	Similar picture to Belladonna, but with less burning of the skin. Headache responds well to cool, open air. Ice-packs to the head may make them feel worse. Head pain accelerates with sunrise, and decreases intensity with sunset. Pains move in an upward direction	Bending head back. Cold applications	Cool, fresh air. Being uncovered. Pressure	Glonoine
Heat exhaustion with cramps	Rapid pulse with nausea, faintness, coldness and pallor. Cramps occur with jerking of muscles ending in possible convulsions. Picture of great weakness and collapse with clammy, profuse sweats	Touch. Motion. Raising arms	Cold drinks	Cuprum
Heat exhaustion with extreme coldness of body and general stiffness	Faintness with heat stroke and rapid pulse and nausea. Sweating is extremely profuse and clammy and accompanied by pallor. Face may be tinged with blue	Touch	Covering. Lying down	Veratrum alb

The following advice will be helpful in addition to selecting the appropriate homoeopathic remedy:

1 Cool the person down as quickly as possible by removing clothing and keeping them in a cool environment. Fanning and cool bathing will also help the cooling process.

2 Rub the limbs vigorously to aid circulation.

3 If the temperature is not dangerously high, drinking a glass of water in which a teaspoonful of salt has been dissolved every half hour for up to three hours will help guard against muscle cramps and dehydration.

4 If there are any signs of unconsciousness developing, treat for shock (see page 39) while sending for help.

5 If the temperature is dangerously high (103° or above) get help as quickly as possible while you attempt to bring the temperature down.

Insect bites and stings

Type	General indications	Worse from	Better for	Remedy name
Marked swelling and puffiness around the bite or sting	Much localised redness, stinging pain, heat, and swelling. Reacts well to cool applications, while pain is made worse by heat. Very useful in cases of Urticaria that develop after a sting	Heat. Touch	Cool bathing. Cool applications	Apis
Bites and stings that feel cold, but are relieved by cold applications	Stinging and pricking pains that are relieved by cool bathing. The area affected by the bite or sting may feel cold to the touch. Lots of swelling and redness accompany discomfort	Warmth	Cold bathing	Ledum
Urticaria which develops after a sting	Stinging and burning pains with raised red blotches. Itching is maddeningly intense	Cool bathing. Touch		Urtica urens
Large and irritating mosquito bites	Stinging, smarting pains accompany mosquito bites. Extreme sensitivity to discomfort	Touch	Warmth. Rest	Staphysagria

If someone is suffering from the effects of a sting, in addition to taking the appropriate homoeopathic remedy, try to remove any sting remaining in the wound and apply cold compresses.

If any of the following occur professional help is needed:

1 Any symptoms of rapidly advancing swelling, especially affecting the mouth and throat.

2 Signs of breathing problems.

3 Confusion, fainting or loss of consciousness.

4 If you have any knowledge that the person affected has a history of allergy to insect or bee/wasp stings.

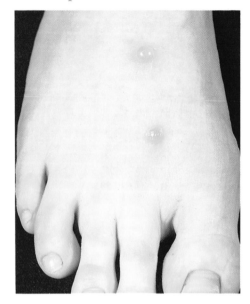

Dental work

Type	General indications	Worse from	Better for	Remedy name
Bruised pain following any dental work except wisdom tooth extractions	Excellent as a first choice of remedy for any work that has caused trauma and bruising to tissue in the mouth. Avoid giving Arnica after extraction of wisdom teeth, since it is so effective at promoting re-absorption of blood, it can lead to a dry socket. In the event of an extraction, choose an alternative appropriate remedy	Least touch		Arnica
Nerve pains following drilling or extraction	Shooting, violent pains that seem to radiate from the point of injury. Often needed if there is discomfort following injection or anaesthetic			Hypericum

Type	General indications	Worse from	Better for	Remedy name
Pains relating to site of injection	Discomfort at the area where injection has been given. Painful area may feel cold, but the pain feels better for cold applications	Heat to painful area	Cold bathing of injured area	Ledum
Deep aching that has not been resolved by using Arnica	Deep aching pains that convey the feeling that bones have been bruised. Often helpful in cases of dry socket. Not likely to be indicated in the early stages following dental work	Cold	Warmth	Ruta
Excessive bleeding following tooth extractions	Profuse bleeding even from a small wound. May be anxious with bleeding and in need of reassurance			Phosphorus
Pains after a filling or extraction with hypersensitivity on both physical and mental levels	Terrific irritability with pain – can't stand exposure to cold in any form. Feels better for warm applications. May be snappy, and just want to be left alone to go to sleep	Cold. Noise. Touch	Napping. Keeping warm	Nux vomica
Severe stitching pains following dental work	Pains are stitching and very severe. Wound feels lacerated with stinging, smarting pains. Feelings of resentment following dental work	Touch. Cold drinks	Warmth. Rest	Staphysagria
Pre-dental work 'nerves'	Terrific feelings of anxiety and fear with awful restlessness. May feel so bad, that death seems preferable to state of nervous tension. Mounting feeling of terror as appointment approaches			Aconite

In addition to selecting the appropriate homoeopathic remedy, the following suggestions may be helpful:

1 Use a mouthwash of Calendula or Hypercal tincture. Dilute 40 drops of tincture in $\frac{1}{4}$ pint of boiled, cooled water and rinse around

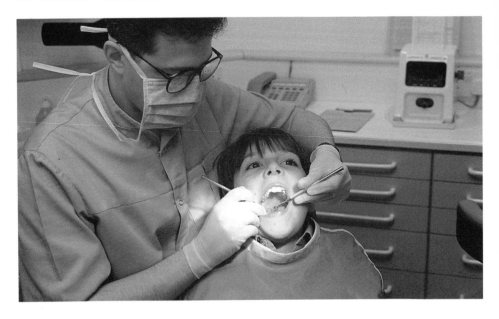

your mouth at regular intervals for a couple of days. This will inhibit infection and speed up healing.

2 If you find a visit to the dentist very traumatic, try to have an afternoon appointment so that you can go home and rest afterwards in order to give your body a chance to recover. Above all, don't force yourself to do something strenuous or demanding if you don't feel up to it.

3 If you have any doubts about the speed it is taking for your mouth to heal, or if pain seems to be continuing for longer than you would expect, do consult your dentist for advice.

Bleeding

Type	General indications	Worse from	Better for	Remedy name
Bleeding following injury	Indicated in bleeding associated with shock or after sustaining an injury. This is one of the first remedies to consider in any trauma state	Least touch	Lying down	Arnica
Bleeding associated with fainting	Bleeding is accompanied by blue-tinged pallor, clammy sweat, and air hunger. The nature of the bleeding is steady and oozing	Warm rooms	Fanning with cool air	Carbo veg

Type	General indications	Worse from	Better for	Remedy name
Bleeding with nauseous sensations, and possible shortness of breath	Bleeding is bright red and comes in spurts or gushes. Symptoms may be accompanied by feeble pulse and cold sweat. Nausea feels much worse for movement	Warmth. Lying down	Open air. Rest	Ipecac
Recurrent nosebleeds or small wounds that bleed profusely	Recurrent nosebleeds that are often sparked off by over-vigorous blowing. Should be considered for any minor wound that bleeds excessively	Touch. Any exertion	Open air. Cold water. Sleep	Phosphorus

In addition to giving the appropriate homoeopathic medicine, try to ensure that bleeding is either stopping or under control.

1 Try direct pressure over the wound (provided it is not a puncture wound where something has remained embedded in it). You should see a reduction in the flow of blood within 15 minutes.

2 Place a sterile dressing over the wound ensuring that it extends beyond the edges. Secure firmly, but not with so much pressure that it interferes with circulation.

3 In nose bleeds, ensure that the patient leans well forward and advise them to breathe through the mouth, while pinching the soft part of the nose. Any blood in the mouth should be spat out to avoid vomiting. If nose bleeds are associated with an injury to the head, get professional advice.

4 If you are in any doubt, always get help as quickly as possible.

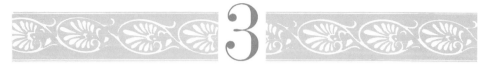

HOMOEOPATHY FOR SORE THROATS, COUGHS AND COLDS

The respiratory system

Breathing is essential to life as it is the process by which we take in oxygen, which is used up by the body, and eliminate the by-product carbon dioxide. Following the path of the air, respiration starts at the nose or mouth where air is breathed in, down the windpipe into the lungs. In the lungs, oxygen is absorbed into the bloodstream to be pumped around the body by the heart. Meanwhile carbon dioxide and water vapour which can't be used by the body are released by the blood into the lungs to be breathed out.

Without the exchange of carbon dioxide and oxygen involved in the process of breathing, life could not be maintained. Seen from this viewpoint, optimum functioning of the respiratory system (the organs and blood involved in the process) is vital to maintaining good health. Short-lived disorders such as the common cold can cause a great deal of discomfort by disrupting the smooth functioning of the respiratory system, and the search for an orthodox medical cure still continues.

Basic drugs used in treating sore throats, coughs and hay fever include antibiotics, cough suppressants or expectorants, and antihistamines. Prophylactic measures are now also adopted such as the administration of a 'flu vaccination before the winter season begins in the hope that it will reduce the number of colds suffered by the patient. The main thrust of the orthodox approach is involved with reducing inflammatory processes which result in fever, mucus production, and general irritation of mucous membranes.

Homoeopathic medicines and the respiratory system

The homoeopathic approach views cold and cough symptoms as the body's mechanism of ridding itself of noxious material. In this light, one can see how mucus discharges are a basic mechanism in flushing toxins out of the body. The coughing reflex can also be seen to be fulfilling the same function as it attempts to expel the by-products of acute infection.

When these processes go on too long, they are unable to carry out their task and result in making the person more and more exhausted and unwell. Instead of attempting to suppress these symptoms, homoeopathic medicines work by giving them a boost and enabling them to carry on the job efficiently and quickly.

For this reason, after an appropriate homoeopathic medicine has been administered, the symptoms occasionally appear to be intensified for a short while as the body rids itself of toxic waste. If this is the result of the homoeopathic medicine, although the symptoms are still present, there will be a general improvement in sense of well-being and vitality. In other words, although the person still has their sore throat or cold, they feel much better in themselves, which is a sign that improvement of the specific symptoms should rapidly follow.

How to select the appropriate homoeopathic medicine

If you have turned to this section of the book because you have just developed the first signs of a cold, this is how you select your homoeopathic remedy:

1 Turn to the table entitled **Colds**, and look down the left hand column entitled **Type** to identify which category your symptoms fall into. If, for example, you have recently been exposed to a chill and started to feel ill soon afterwards, the chances are that the column entitled 'Early stage, after exposure to dry, cold winds' is likely to be most useful.

2 Check with the **General indications** in the next column that these symptoms fit with your own. If you have lots of sneezing, feel thirsty, and generally seem anxious and restless since the symptoms developed, it looks like you are still on the right track. If, on the other hand, you have a high temperature, look flushed and generally feel feverish and irritable, take a look at the other early onset remedies such as Belladonna and Ferrum phos. Remember that you are looking for the general symptom picture that most clearly matches your own.

3 Finally check the **Worse from** and **Better for** columns to see if these also fit. Do bear in mind that these two columns do not just refer to what makes your cold symptoms feel better or worse, but also what might make you generally feel better or worse. So, if, for example, you have definitely noticed that you feel much worse at night, or from being in a warm room, but feel better from fresh air, the chances are that Aconite will be the best remedy for you.

4 Remember that a cold generally passes through a number of different stages before it resolves itself, and that you are likely to need a change of remedy at each stage. In other words, once you have passed the stage of initial onset, Aconite is no longer likely to be appropriate to your symptoms. Just take note of any changes, e.g. if you begin to develop a cough, and use the same method described above to find what the most appropriate remedy is likely to be. You may also combine tables (e.g. if you have both a sore throat and cough at the same time) always remembering that you are looking for the single homoeopathic remedy that covers the whole symptom picture most adequately.

5 It is unlikely that a homoeopathic remedy would abort a cold, but if the selection of remedy is appropriate, it will take you through the various stages quickly, and with the minimum amount of discomfort.

For information on how to take the appropriate remedy, see the section entitled **How to take homoeopathic medicines** in the chapter on **Practical Homoeopathy**; exactly the same principles apply.

Sore throats/tonsilitis

Type	General indications	Worse from	Better for	Remedy name
Sore throat with high fever	Very bright red throat with lots of pain trying to swallow liquids. Aversion to drinking. 'Strawberry' tongue (covered with bright red spots). Dry mouth and throat. Pains may extend to right ear on swallowing. Generally red, flushed, and feverish	Drinking. Talking. Empty swallowing	Rest in bed	Belladonna (most useful in the first 24 hours)
Sore throat with fear and anxiety	Sore throat may come on after exposure to cold or draughts. Fever may be high with fear and restlessness. Inflammation of throat with stitching pains. Desire to swallow which aggravates feeling of constriction and pain	Extreme changes from heat or cold. At night	Open air. Sleep	Aconite (most useful in first 24 hours)
Sore throat with extreme swelling	Glossy, 'water-bag' (look as though filled with water) appearance to the throat, tonsils, and tongue. Pains are characteristically stinging and hot	Warm drinks. Touch	Cold drinks. Cold surround-ings	Apis

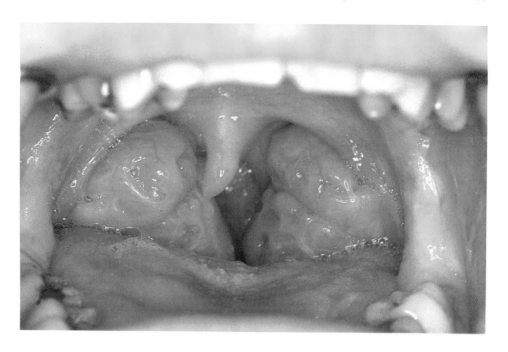

Sore throats/tonsilitis (established stage)

Type	General indications	Worse from	Better for	Remedy name
Left-sided pain with lots of constriction	Pain often starts on the left side and extends to the ear. Difficulty swallowing because of a sensation of a lump in the throat. Possible ulceration of the throat. Dislikes having anything constricting around the neck	After sleep. Empty swallowing. Warm drinks. Warm rooms	Swallowing food. Cold drinks. Open air	Lachesis
Sore throat with painful, inflamed glands	Ulcerated throat with offensive breath and lots of saliva in the mouth. Pains may begin on the right hand side and move to the left. Very restless and aggravated by extremes of temperature. May be very sweaty	At night. Heat of the bed. Cold surround-ings	Regular temperature	Merc sol

Type	General indications	Worse from	Better for	Remedy name
Sore throat with aching pains in the body	Generally feels unwell and feverish. Lots of glandular unease and shooting pains to the ears on swallowing. Severe inflammation of the throat that looks very dark red or purple in colour. Very chilly, even when covered. Pain at base of tongue when extended	Hot drinks. Right side. Cold	Warmth	Phytolacca
Sore throat with sharp, splinter-like pains	Very toxic conditions with tendency to pus formation. Ulceration of the throat with a sensation as though there were a fish bone or splinter embedded in it. Shooting pains extending to the ears when not swallowing. Irritability and hypersensitivity with illness. Strong dislike of being cold	Cold in any form	Warmth	Hepar sulph
Sore throat which begins on the right and moves to the left	Generally slow onset of feeling unwell or malaise. Sensation of lump rising in the throat with constant desire to swallow. Symptoms in general may be aggravated mid-afternoon until early evening	Cold drinks. Heat of room. At night	Warm drinks. Open air	Lycopodium

Laryngitis

Type	General indications	Worse from	Better for	Remedy name
Sudden loss of voice from exposure to dry, cold winds	Loss of voice with fever, anxiety and restlessness. May accompany croupy cough in children	Exposure to cold air. At night	Sleep	Aconite

Type	General indications	Worse from	Better for	Remedy name
Dry, sore throat with loss of voice	Hoarseness or complete loss of voice with constant desire to clear the throat. Much worse on attempting to speak. Throat feels very dry and sensitive to touch or cold air Dry, tickling cough may accompany loss of voice	Evening. Talking. Cold air	Sound sleep. Reassurance. Cool drinks	Phosphorus
Loss of voice from emotional upset or shock	Sensation of lump in the throat with constriction. May feel throat is constantly sore since grief or shock	Dry swallowing. Fluids	Swallowing food. Distraction	Ignatia

Once you have selected the most appropriate homoeopathic remedy, the following suggestions may be useful as supportive measures in order to speed up the natural healing process:

1 Take plenty of fluids to keep the temperature down and flush toxins out of the body. Mineral water tends to be best suited to this purpose rather than warm drinks like coffee or tea which encourage dehydration.

2 Vitamin C may be useful as a supplement to assist the immune system in fighting the infection. Between 1–3 grams may be taken in a 24 hour period for one to three days. Always reduce the amount of vitamin C taken if diarrhoea occurs, since this is a sign that a lower dose is needed. Once the reduction has been made digestion should return to normal.

3 Avoid foods which are painful to swallow and difficult to digest. Home-made soups and steamed vegetables, fruit or salads are likely to be most digestible, nutritious, and easy on the throat.

4 Try to rest as much as possible to aid the body in fighting infection.

5 Avoid moving from one extreme of temperature to another and try to humidify the air by placing containers of water at strategic places, e.g. near radiators.

6 Gargle with a solution of warm water and salt or lemon and honey. A very soothing gargle may also be made by diluting Hypercal tincture (a mixture of Hypericum and Calendula tincture) in warm water.

If any of the following occur, professional help should be considered:

1 If throat pain is severe with difficulty swallowing.

2 Sore throats in children with fever which looks persistent.

3 A sore throat in anyone who has suffered from rheumatic fever.

4 Sore throats accompanied by a rash and a high temperature.

5 Ulceration or pus formation in the throat.

6 Any problems with breathing or drooling accompanying a sore throat should be investigated quickly.

Colds

Type	General indications	Worse from	Better for	Remedy name
Early stage with high temperature	Very hot and feverish with dry, bright red skin. Symptoms come on rapidly and progress quickly. Very restless and irritable. Pulse may be rapid	Light. Noise. Motion	Sitting upright in bed	Belladonna
Early stage after exposure to dry, cold winds	Very restless with strong anxiety. Lots of sneezing with dry sensations in the nose or fluent nasal discharge in the mornings. Throat and chest feel sore and constricted. Thirsty for large quantities of water. Colds may develop after fright or shock	Night. Warm room. Talking	Open air	Aconite
Early stage of cold with shivering, chills and feverish feelings	Not so intensely hot as Belladonna, or as anxious as Aconite. Hot face with well-defined circular patches on cheeks. May feel generally heavy and weary	Night. Cold air	Warmth. Cold applications	Ferrum phos
Colds with lots of sneezing and streaming eyes and nose	Streaming eyes and nose accompany sneezing. Discharges are burning, profuse and watery. Red, burning and inflamed eyes with bland discharge. Nasal discharge burns top lip	Warm rooms. Indoors. Evening	Out of doors. Cool rooms	Allium cepa

Type	General indications	Worse from	Better for	Remedy name
Colds with profuse nasal discharge and tears	Fluent, bland nasal discharge with copious burning tears (the complete opposite of Allium cepa). Chilly with frequent sneezing and light sensitivity	Night. Lying down. Open air. Light	During the day	Euphrasia
Colds with extreme physical and mental irritability and sensitivity	Slow onset of cold after exposure to dry, cold weather. Lots of sneezing and tickling in the nose, with itching in the ears. Nose runs in warm room and during the day, but feels stuffed up at night. Lots of irritability and physical sensitivity to draughts of cold air	Eating. On waking. Cold air. Mental exertion. Lack of sleep	Warmth. Napping	Nux vomica
Colds with cold sores and dry lips	Lots of nasal discharge which looks like raw egg white. Loss of smell and taste with post-nasal drip. Lips may be cracked in the centre. May be depressed with cold symptoms, but aggravated by sympathy and attention	Sympathy. Sunlight. Warmth. After sleep	Open air. Not eating	Nat mur

For general advice on adjunctive way of dealing with cold symptoms see Influenza section.

Influenza ('flu)

Type	General indications	Worse from	Better for	Remedy name
Rapid onset of symptoms with high temperature	Rapid pulse with very bright red, dry, hot skin. Throbbing pains which are made worse by any movement. This remedy is likely to be of most use within the first 24 hours of symptoms developing	Motion. Stimulation. Light. Noise	Lying semi-upright in bed	Belladonna

Type	General indications	Worse from	Better for	Remedy name
'Flu symptoms with exhaustion and anxiety	Extreme restlessness and anxiety over symptoms. Lots of burning pains which are better for heat (except headache which may respond better to fresh air). Very chilly with a desire for warmth. Responds well to company and distraction	Night. Food. Cold	Warmth. Company. Rest. Open air	Arsenicum album
Classic 'flu symptoms with shivering, aching, and fatigue	Slow onset with chills running up and down spine. Feels very heavy and lethargic with general aches and pains. May have high temperature without thirst. Withdrawn and apathetic	Change of climate. Motion	Urination. Alcohol. Open air	Gelsemium
'Flu with extreme weakness and aching deep in the bones	Deep aching pains in the back and limbs, bones feel as if they were broken. Desire to keep still because of the degree of pain. Chilly and feverish with bursting headache. Eyes may feel particularly aching and sore. Bilious feelings with 'flu	Cold air. Moving	Distraction. Warmth	Eupatorium perfoliatum
'Flu with stiff and aching muscles – much worse at night	May come on after exposure to damp cold weather. Glands are swollen, hard and painful. Cannot find any position in bed at night that affords any relief. Nose may be congested with thick, green mucus. Chilly feelings alternate with flushes of heat	Night. Cold air. Rest	Warmth. Gentle movement	Rhus tox

Type	General indications	Worse from	Better for	Remedy name
Established stage of 'flu symptoms with stubborn catarrhal symptoms	Changeability of symptoms. Weepiness and feelings of depression with illness which are improved by consolation and attention. Mucus discharges are bland, thick and greeny-yellow. May have discomfort in sinuses and glands. Chilly, but feels better for fresh air	Stuffy rooms. Rest. After eating	Cool air. Gentle motion. Crying	Pulsatilla

The following measures may be helpful in addition to selecting the appropriate homoeopathic remedy:

1 Stay in as even a temperature as possible, especially if you suspect your temperature may be high. Moving from one extreme to another is only likely to make you feel worse.

2 It is very important to rest as much as possible to allow the body as much chance as possible to fight the infection. This takes energy, so it is a very good idea not to make any extra demands on your body to allow the natural healing process to take place.

3 Useful supplements include vitamin C and Garlic Pearles which are both thought to aid in mobilising the body's own defences in dealing with infection. Try 1–3 grams of vitamin C daily for two to three days, depending on bowel tolerance, cutting down the dosage until the digestion settles down. Two Garlic Pearles may be taken three times a day for as long as the infection continues.

4 Keep your diet as light as possible and drink as much water as you can to help your body flush out toxins and loosen mucus. Drinking fluids regularly becomes a strong priority if you have a raised temperature.

If any of the following occur you should consider professional help:

1 Raised temperature in a baby or young child.

2 Raised temperature accompanied by stiff neck, lethargy, irritability, and changed breathing.

3 Stubborn raised temperature in otherwise fit adults that does not respond to naturopathic or homoeopathic measures.

4 If in doubt get help. It is always better to err on the cautious side, especially where young children or elderly people are concerned since illnesses can develop rapidly at both sides of the age spectrum.

Coughs

Type	General indications	Worse from	Better for	Remedy name
Early stage of cough after exposure to dry, cold winds	Croupy-sounding cough that is particularly disturbing in the later part of the night. Lots of anxiety and restlessness with coughing bouts. Cough may sound barking and choking	Exposure to cold. Talking. Smoke	Warm rooms. Lying down	Aconite
Dry cough with wheezing, especially bad at night	Lots of restlessness and anxiety with cough, especially marked at night. Cough is dry and tickling making the person sit up in bed at night for relief. Cough is aggravated from exposure to cold, and relieved by sips of warm drinks. Burning pains in the chest with wheezing	Cold. Night. Exertion	Warmth. Lying with head elevated. Company	Arsenicum album
Dry, irritating cough with desire to press on the chest	Hard, dry cough which is made worse entering a warm room. May have marked thirst for large quantities of cold water. Headache may accompany the cough. Pains in the chest from coughing are relieved by firm pressure, either by lying on the painful area, or pressing the hand firmly against it	Eating. Drinking. Warm rooms. Taking a deep breath	Pressure. Fresh air. Lying still	Bryonia
Exhausting cough with hoarseness which is much worse for talking	Head colds which descend to the chest causing a tickly, burning cough which exhausts. Mucus discharges are characteristically yellow-green in colour or containing streaks of blood. May be called for in the early stages of bronchitis. Chest may feel tight and heavy	Changes of temperature. Moving. Talking. Cold drinks	Company. Attention. Sleep	Phos

Type	General indications	Worse from	Better for	Remedy name
Cough with gagging and retching	Nature of the cough resembles Whooping Cough. Bouts of coughing follow each other in close succession. Coughing bouts end in retching. Coughing characteristically comes soon as the person lies down	Lying down. Eating and drinking	Keeping chest still. Open air	Drosera
Dry, shallow cough with extreme sensitivity to cold air	Cough set off by breathing in cold air and relieved by staying in constant temperature. Barking, hacking cough which prevents sleep. Cough aggravated by talking and touching the external throat	Cold air. Changes of temperature. Lying down	Warm air	Rumex crispus
Cough which is so hard and rasping, it sounds like a saw being drawn through dry wood	Dryness of mucus membranes with severe barking cough. Larynx feels obstructed, burning and dry. May be woken from sleep by suffocating sensations accompanying the cough	Very cold drinks. After sleep. Dry, cold wind	Eating or drinking a little. Warmth	Spongia
Established state of cough with copious yellow-green mucus discharges	Cough may alternate between being dry at night, and loose during the day and on waking. Characteristic dry mouth without thirst, and chilliness with desire for open air may accompany the cough. Generally feels better for gentle motion out of doors. May be depressed and weepy with the cough	Stuffy rooms. Keeping still	Sitting up in bed. Open air. Gentle exercise. Sympathy	Pulsatilla

Type	General indications	Worse from	Better for	Remedy name
Cough with brassy sound and stubborn, tough mucus	Tickling sensation at the base of the throat that precedes cough. Lots of stringy, ropy, tough mucus that may be difficult to dislodge. Mucus deposits may lead to sinus pain at the root of the nose. Most likely to be of use in the later stages of a head cold that has travelled downwards	Eating. Damp cold. After sleep. Open air	Heat. Bringing up mucus	Kali bich

General advice for coughs will be basically the same as advice already given in the section on Colds and Influenza with the addition of the following.

1 Avoid milk and milk products if you have a cough since these foods are mucus-forming and can aggravate a cough, especially if taken before bed time.

2 Try to avoid dry atmospheres by placing containers of water near sources of heat, or making use of a commercially manufactured humidifier. If coughing is particularly troublesome, spending some time in a steam-filled bathroom may help breathing temporarily.

If any of the following occur professional help may be needed:

1 If wheezing occurs in someone who has not experienced this before.

2 Marked chest pain.

3 Accelerated breathing or breathing difficulties, especially in young children.

4 If you suspect any foreign body has been inhaled.

5 Any signs of confusion or drowsiness.

6 If a cough has persisted with no observable improvement and accompanied by a general decline in energy and well-being.

Sinusitis

Type	General indications	Worse from	Better for	Remedy name
Sinus pain made worse by touch or exposure to cold	Very sensitive to even the slightest draught of cold air. Also very irritable and emotionally sensitive. Pain may be concentrated at the base of the nose, and the whole skull may feel bruised	Cold. Touch. Dry winds	Heat. Moist air	Hepar sulph
Pain and congestion located specifically at the root of the nose	Lots of nasal mucus which is very tough and stringy. General soreness in facial bones, with shooting pains in the sinuses in the region of the cheeks. Pulsating pains and dryness of mucus membranes	Stooping. Damp weather. Cold weather. Motion	Warmth. Pressure	Kali bich
Sinus pains improved by wrapping up firmly	Pains often come on after getting wet and chilled. There may be hard, crusting in the nose and at the meeting places of mucus membranes and skin. Pains are markedly improved by exertion of pressure to the painful spot	Cold. Noise. Motion. Talking	Warmth.	Silica
Sinus pain from long-standing catarrhal conditions with bland, yellow-green mucus	Loss of smell with sinus pains. Nose is stuffed up in the evening and night, but mucus flows more freely in the morning. Nose also feels more stuffed up in warm rooms, and feels more comfortable out of doors. Weepiness and desire for sympathy may accompany sinus symptoms	Stuffy rooms. At night. Heat	Open air. Gentle motion. Cold in general	Pulsatilla

Type	General indications	Worse from	Better for	Remedy name
Sinus pains which are raw and burning with offensive nasal discharges	Pressured feeling in bones of the face with sensation of swelling inside the nose. Thin nasal discharges changing to thick offensive mucus. Marked increase in amount of saliva in the mouth, tongue may seem swollen. Generally feels chilly and sweaty	At night. Extreme temperature changes. Draught	Moderate temperature. Rest	Merc sol

Follow the general suggestions in the sections above to help deal with inflamed sinuses.

If the following occur, it is worth considering professional help:

1 High temperature and/or offensive nasal discharges accompanying sinus pain.

2 If pain is severe and fails to respond to homoeopathic treatment in approximately 24 hours.

Hay fever

While the following may be useful in giving acute relief during the summer season for hay fever symptoms, it is recommended that long-term homoeopathic treatment from a trained practitioner is sought in order to deal with the predisposition to the condition.

Type	General indications	Worse from	Better for	Remedy name
Hay fever symptoms with extreme swelling and puffiness	Eyes and throat are exceptionally red and puffy. Swellings look like water bags and are accompanied by stinging pains. Symptoms are generally strongly aggravated by heat and improved by cold	Heat. Touch. Lying down	Cold air and cold bathing	Apis

Type	General indications	Worse from	Better for	Remedy name
Hay fever accompanied by burning, scanty mucus discharges	Lots of burning accompanying scanty, clear nasal discharge. Responds better to warmth than cold. May feel very anxious and restless with symptoms. Eyes are likely to be watery and very sensitive to light with peripheral swelling	Cold. Outside. Night	Warmth. Inside. Rest	Arsenicum album
Hay fever with profuse, clear discharges	Frequent, violent sneezing with accompanying profuse watery discharges from eyes and nose. May develop cold sores after exposure to sunlight, or cracked lips	Sunlight. Warmth. Exertion. Sympathy	Open air. Cool. Being left alone	Natrum mur
Hay fever with extreme sensitivity on both physical and emotional levels	Terrific sensitivity to draughts of cold air, light and odours. Eyes may be bloodshot and watery, and sneezing is likely to be violent and frequent, especially on waking. Very irritable and bad-tempered which is worse early on the day, but gets better as the day goes on	Odours. Stimulation. Early in the day. Cold air	Damp weather. Warmth. In the evening	Nux vomica
Hay fever with very bland, thick discharges	Blocked nasal passages feel much worse indoors, especially in a stuffy room. Generally improved by being in the open air. Nose blocks at night, and runs more fluently in the day. May feel chilly, but still desires to be out of doors	Warmth. Night. Rest	Open air. Gentle motion. Consolation. Cold applications	Pulsatilla
Hay fever with bland discharges from eyes, but acrid discharge from nasal passages	Lots of sneezing with profuse, bland discharge from eyes which smart. Burning of the upper lip from thin, watery discharge from nose	Warmth. Damp weather	Cool, open air. Motion	Allium cepa

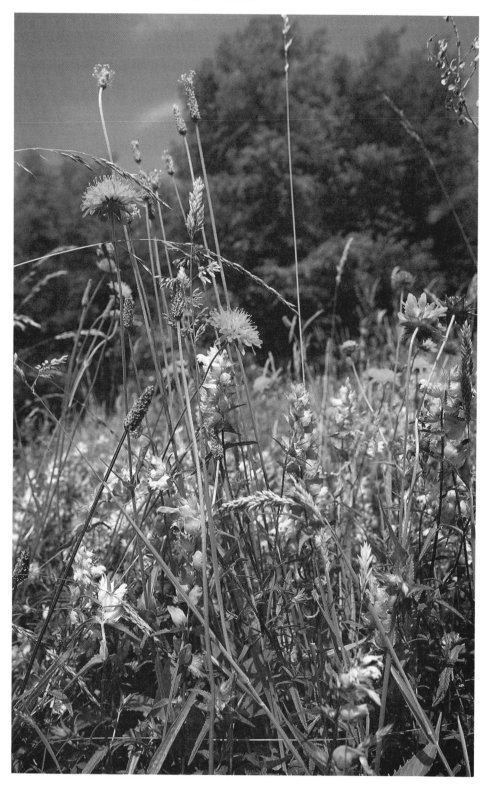

Type	General indications	Worse from	Better for	Remedy name
Hay fever with bland nasal discharge, and acrid tears from eyes	Profuse, hot, acrid tears which require frequent wiping. Eyes are very bloodshot and sensitive to light. Lots of bland nasal mucus with possible chest involvement	Sunlight. Wind. Warm rooms	Open air. Wiping eyes	Euphrasia
Hay fever with very persistent sneezing which may be abortive	Intense itching in nose with strong desire to rub it. Tickling sensation in nose may spread over whole body. Extremely sensitive sense of smell with single nostril blocked at one time. Nasal discharge increases even at the thought of the smell of flowers	Cold air. Strong odours. Mental exertion	Open air. Warmth. Eating	Sabadilla

The following measures may be helpful in soothing symptoms:

1 Rinse eyes and nasal passages with sterile water.

2 Inhaling steam may help open swollen airways.

3 Increase your fluid intake (preferably water).

4 Avoid obvious substances which are likely to irritate your allergy further such as dust, perfume or animal hair.

General advice

With disorders of the respiratory system such as colds and sore throats, it is worth saying that it is not always necessary to prescribe homoeopathic medicines to get over the condition. Very often, the general hints given at the end of each section are enough on their own to make you sufficiently comfortable to get over the illness speedily and well. If, on the other hand, while you are following the general advice, the symptoms are making you feel very unwell, prescribing the appropriate homoeopathic medicine at the right time will help enormously in speeding up the healing process and improving your general sense of well-being.

4

HOMOEOPATHY FOR DIGESTIVE UPSETS

The digestive system

Looked at from a mechanistic standpoint, the digestive system is a food processing machine which opens at one end with the mouth and ends at the other with the anus. In between there are organs which perform certain functions like the stomach, liver, and intestines which break down the ingested food into useful or discardable components.

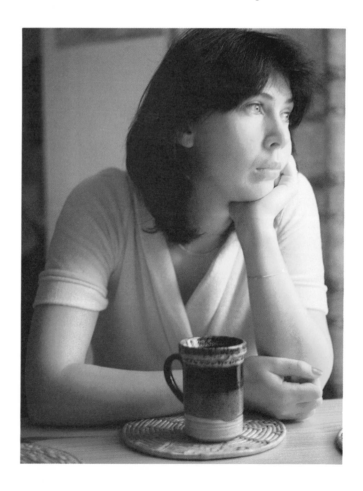

If something goes wrong with this system, the orthodox medical approach involves using drugs to suppress the specific system, thus providing a mechanical answer to the problem. In other words, if the problem with the digestive system involves the secretion of too much acid in the stomach, an antacid is used to dilute the stomach secretions temporarily. Or if constipation arises, a laxative is given to stimulate the bowel to evacuate itself more frequently. From these examples it is obvious that orthodox medical drugs work from the premise that when a digestive problem arises, it is that particular compartment of the body which is malfunctioning and requires a mechanical adjustment.

Homoeopathic medicines and the digestive system

Homoeopathic medical theory approaches the concept of disease from a different perspective. Rather than viewing symptoms of illness as an indication that one part alone of the body is in trouble, symptoms are seen as indicators that the whole body has shifted into a state of imbalance. This is particularly relevant to a discussion of digestive problems, since many people experience nausea or acid indigestion as part of an overall systemic response to stress or an overburdened lifestyle.

The most basic concept in homoeopathic theory is that, when well, (i.e. in a state of balance), the human body is capable of carrying out all its necessary functions without the help of drugs, because of the presence of biochemical checks and balances which maintain the smooth functioning of the various systems within the body. When stresses occur which knock this self-regulatory functioning off balance, symptoms appear. These are the first indications that all is not well. When the required homoeopathic medicine is given at this stage, the body regains its equilibrium and bodily functions are regulated once more to their original smooth functioning.

How to select the appropriate homoeopathic medicine

If you have turned to this section of the book because you are in the throes of a digestive problem like indigestion, this is how you select your homoeopathic remedy:

1 Turn to the table entitled **Indigestion**, and look down the left hand column entitled **Type** to identify which category your symptoms fall into. If, for example, your stomach normally functions very well, but you have had terrible indigestion since you have been given a date for your driving test, the chances are that the column entitled 'Indigestion from anticipation' is the one for you.

2 Check with the **General indications** that these symptoms fit with your own. If you have acid burping and lots of rumbling and gurgling with bloating, then it definitely looks like you are on the right track.

3 Finally check the **Worse from** and **Better for** columns to see if these also fit. Do bear in mind that these two columns do not just refer

to what makes your indigestion better or worse, but also what might make you *generally* feel better or worse. So, if you have definitely noticed that you feel much worse after eating, but warm drinks or loosening your clothes help your indigestion, the chances are that Lycopodium is the remedy for you.

4 You will find some suggestions at the end of the section on Indigestion of general ways of preventing the condition recurring once you have been helped by the indicated remedy.

For information on how to take the appropriate remedy, see the section entitled **How to take homoeopathic medicines** in the chapter on **Practical Homoeopathy**; exactly the same principles apply.

Indigestion

Type	General indications	Worse from	Better for	Remedy name
Indigestion with bloating and excess wind	Extreme swelling around the waist which is much worse after eating anything. Heavy and full sensations in the stomach, with violent burping	Stuffy rooms. Tight clothes	Fresh air. Passing wind	Carbo veg
Indigestion from anticipation	Bloating with noisy rumbling and gurgling in stomach and abdomen. Eating very little makes the stomach feel full. Acid burping	Eating a large amount. Tight clothes	Warm drinks	Lycopodium
Indigestion from fatty, rich foods	Indigestion may follow an overly-indigestible meal with lots of red meat or cheese. The mouth may be dry with no thirst, and 'repeating' of food eaten hours before. Weepiness may accompany indigestion	Stuffy rooms. Resting	Fresh air. Gentle movement. Cold drinks	Pulsatilla

Type	General indications	Worse from	Better for	Remedy name
'Morning after' indigestion	A classic hangover headache may accompany the indigestion. Aching may be felt across the eyes or at the back of the head. Sour-tasting burps which are difficult to bring up. Irritability of mind and body	Any effort. Too little sleep	Napping. Resting	Nux vomica
Acid indigestion from anxiety	Much burning in the stomach relieved by small sips of cold water or tea. Feelings of anxious restlessness with nausea. Prostrated with feelings of sickness. May be chilly with nausea	Any physical exertion. Being chilly	Keeping warm. Resting	Arsenicum album

Once you have gained relief from a well-chosen homoeopathic remedy, the following measures will help prevent the condition occurring again.

1 Eating slowly and trying to relax during a meal are very important ways of preventing indigestion occurring. Eating is a very sensual experience since more senses than taste alone are brought into play. Lots of people are unaware that digestive juices begin to flow from just smelling and seeing appetising food, so that the process of digestion can begin long before you put any food into your mouth. Also remember that your stomach is made of muscle, and, like any other muscular structure, can suffer from tension. If your stomach muscles are in a state of tension when food enters the stomach, the wave-like muscular contractions called peristalsis can't happen smoothly. Peristalsis is responsible for smooth digestion, and if it is hampered, the chances are that pain and gas will be the result.

2 Some foods have a bad reputation for contributing to indigestion and are best avoided if you feel an attack developing. The best known foods in this category are raw onions, peppers, cabbage, and beans. Common irritants of the stomach lining include strong coffee, tea, curries, chillies, and smoking. Very fatty foods like full fat cheese, cream and red meat and pork are probably also best avoided if you're feeling queasy.

3 If indigestion or heartburn are persistent and troublesome over a period of time, seek professional help.

Vomiting and diarrhoea

Type	General indications	Worse from	Better for	Remedy name
Food poisoning (1)	Vomiting and diarrhoea which occur simultaneously after eating spoiled food. Exhaustion with vomiting to the point of collapse. General sense of chilliness which responds well to warmth. Burning pains relieved by warmth. Restless and anxious with vomiting and diarrhoea	Cold. Night. Being alone	Resting. Warmth (apart from head pain which is relieved by cold)	Arsenicum album
Food poisoning (2)	Extreme pallor of the face with profuse, chilly sweat. Alternating vomiting and diarrhoea. Chilly but responds well to cool, fresh air. Vomiting is very violent and projectile, preceded by strong feelings of nausea. Overwhelming thirst for cool drinks	Movement. Warmth. Night	Rest. Cool drinks. Lying down	Veratrum album
Severe nausea with vomiting	Constant nausea that is not relieved by vomiting. Colicky pains with tender, bloated abdomen. Constant sensation of needing to empty the bowels, with nausea. Irritable and oversensitive	Extreme cold or heat. Movement	Rest. Open air	Ipecac
Profuse, violent diarrhoea	Constant painless diarrhoea. Lots of gurgling in bowels. If vomiting occurs with diarrhoea the whole abdomen may feel sore	Early morning. Hot weather. Milk	Rubbing the painful area. Lying on the stomach	Podo-phyllum

Type	General indications	Worse from	Better for	Remedy name
Upset stomachs from 'exam nerves'	'Butterflies' in the stomach with excitement. Loss of appetite with queasy feelings in the stomach. Nervous diarrhoea passed without pain. Withdrawn with anxiety	Anticipation. Worry	Relaxation	Gelsemium
Diarrhoea from fear or excitement	Nausea relieved by eating which makes the stomach pains worse. Nausea relieved by sour things. Craving for sugar which aggravates. Noisy belching and severe diarrhoea aggravated by eating sweets. Talkative and exhuberant from 'nerves'	Anxiety. Closed-in places. Sugar	Cool, open air. Motion. Passing wind	Argentum nit

In addition to selecting the most appropriate homoeopathic remedy, the following suggestions may be helpful in cases of vomiting and diarrhoea.

1 If vomiting and/or diarrhoea occur, the chances are that the digestive tract is attempting to deal with an infection by expelling the contents of the stomach and bowel. In this situation, trying to put more food into the digestive system is counter-productive, so it is best to avoid eating while the vomiting and diarrhoea continue. Once things have settled, go back to eating slowly, avoiding any oils, milk, or other fats. The best thing to begin with would be a little brown rice with lightly-steamed easily digested vegetables, or a little broth.

2 Although eating is a bad idea during vomiting and diarrhoea, drinking is essential to ensure that the body does not get dehydrated. Large quantities of fluid are lost from the body when diarrhoea and vomiting occur together, so check with the signs listed below if you feel dehydration may be a problem. The best fluid to drink is plain water; avoid milk and orange juice which will only irritate the digestive tract further.

If any of the following symptoms occur it would be advisable to get professional help:

1 Any abdominal pain which is persistent, especially if it is accompanied by tenderness, vomiting, diarrhoea, or slightly raised temperature.

2 Persistent vomiting or diarrhoea, especially if there is any presence of blood in the vomit or stools.

3 Signs of dehydration, especially in the very young or elderly:
Skin which looses elasticity (pinch a little skin on the back of the hand; if it doesn't spring back into shape quickly, check for other signs of dehydration);
Lack of saliva or tears;

Sunken fontanelle in babies (located at the crown of the head);
Reduced urine output;
Sunken eyes.

4 Any vomiting or nausea following a head injury.

Constipation

Type	General indications	Worse from	Better for	Remedy name
Constipation with hangover	General irritability and headache accompany constipation. Useful after abuse of drugs like painkillers and over-use of laxatives. Lots of straining and fruitless urging. Never feels finished – incomplete passage of stool	Eating. Broken sleep. Stimulants	Rest. Sleep	Nux vomica
Constipation without any urge to go	No desire to pass stool – total feeling of inactivity in bowel. Stool is uncomfortably large, very dark, dry, and painful to pass. Large thirst for cold drinks. Irritability and headache with constipation	Heat. Effort	Cold drinks. Being still	Bryonia
Constipation with soft, difficult stool	Difficulty passing sticky stools because of inactivity of the bowel. Stool will either be excessively soft, or hard and knotted. Itching and burning of anus with constipation	Sitting still	Eating. Warmth	Alumina
Constipation with anal fissure	Several days may go by with no urging, but once stool is passed it consists of small balls covered with mucus. Aching in rectum after passage of stool	Cold. Over-heating. Before and after periods	Rest. Open air	Graphites

Type	General indications	Worse from	Better for	Remedy name
Constipation away from home	Habitual constipation on holiday. Lots of fruitless urging with noisy wind and bloating. May feel anxiety about being constipated	Travel. Tight clothes. Eating	Warm drinks	Lycopodium

Once the acute situation has been dealt with homoeopathically, the following advice will help prevent the situation occurring again.

1 Have a good look at your diet since, in many cases, constipation can be rectified or significantly improved by making certain dietary changes. Reduce foods which contain lots of white flour and sugar, also try to ensure that dietary fat (butter, cheese, milk and eggs) makes up no more than 20 per cent of your total intake.

It is best to put the emphasis on raw fruit and vegetables, wholemeal bread, and other foods naturally high in fibre like lentils and beans.

Try also to drink enough water. This sounds obvious, but many people do not realise that tea and coffee are no substitutes for water as a lubricant to the digestive system. Try to drink a minimum of four or five glasses of water a day.

2 It is best to avoid cooking with aluminium pans or using tea bags, which also use aluminium in the manufacturing process. Traces of aluminium in the diet can contribute to constipation, as well as a host of other problems, including slow learning in the young, exacerbation of osteoporosis (brittle bones), and deterioration of the brain.

3 Always try to act on the urge to pass a stool (provided of course it's socially acceptable!). Ignoring these important signals can be the first step to developing a problem with constipation.

4 It is best to avoid depending on laxatives to achieve a regular bowel movement, since the formation of this habit can lead to an ultimate aggravation of the problem by making the bowel become progressively more 'lax'. It is also very easy to get into a pattern of alternation of constipation with a form of diarrhoea promoted by the over-use of laxatives: this can lead in the end to problems of malabsorption, where essential nutrients are not given the chance to be utilised by the body.

If you notice any of the following you may benefit from professional advice:

1 If you experience a marked change in your bowel habit for a period of time which is not attributable to a change in diet or routine.

2 Signs of blood in stools especially if it is dark in colour.

Haemorrhoids

Type	General indications	Worse from	Better for	Remedy name
Haemorrhoids with sharp pains and swelling	Sensations as though rectum was full of sharp sticks after passing stool. Swollen sensation in rectum, and pains that persist for several hours	Walking. Bending	Cool	Aescalus hippocastanum
Bluish haemorrhoids with burning pains	Haemorrhoids that resemble a bunch of grapes in appearance. Bearing-down pains with burning, relieved by moving about	Sitting	Bathing with cool water. Moving about	Aloes
Haemorrhoids with shooting pains	Pains are stinging, burning, and shoot upwards. Lots of itching in anus after passing stool	Eating starch. Warmth of bed	Resting	Alumina
Excessively sensitive haemorrhoids	Full sensation in haemorrhoids with constricted sensation in rectum. Bruised pains with stitching sensations radiating up spine. Easy-bleeding haemorrhoids	Exertion. Alcohol and coffee	Resting. Warmth	Nux vomica
Haemorrhoids with chronically inactive bowels	Painful sensitivity in rectum for hours after passing unusually large, hard, dry stool. No urge to go at all	Warmth. Moving	Resting. Cool	Bryonia
Bleeding haemorrhoids	Sensations of bruised soreness with bleeding from the rectum. Haemorrhoids feel tense or bursting. Affected area feels swollen and inflamed	Pressure. Jarring. Touch		Hamamelis

The pain and discomfort of haemorrhoids can be significantly eased by judicious use of homoeopathic medicines. The following hints may also be useful in helping to deal with more deep-seated underlying factors which may be aggravating the condition.

1 Try to evaluate the quality of your diet, bearing in mind the advice already given in the Constipation section. There is not

much point in trying to ease the discomfort of haemorrhoids if your diet is causing habitual straining and constipation.

2 You may find a homoeopathic cream useful to soothe the painful area from without as well as using homoeopathic remedies internally. Companies such as Nelsons market creams especially suited to this purpose. These should be available in health food shops and chemists stocking homoeopathic remedies.

3 It is also worth trying a warm bath before applying a soothing cream if haemorrhoids are inflamed and painful.

Beyond the immediate problem: general advice on digestion

All of us know by now about the value of exercise and its role in stress reduction, but perhaps fewer of us realise how helpful regular exercise can be to the healthy functioning of the digestive organs.

Apart from having a beneficial effect on stress levels (which has its own spin-off effect on digestion), regular exercise can help a great deal with a digestive problem like constipation. Lots of people suffer irregular bowel movements because of the lack of tone of their bowels which can result from sitting in an office all day. This is a problem which can be further compounded by a bad diet, or just sheer lack of time for eating regular meals.

When choosing an exercise programme, bear in mind that it needs to be one that suits your temperament. If exercise isn't enjoyable and fun, then the chances are that it will become a chore which only adds more stress to your life. Also try to aim for regularity rather than having long

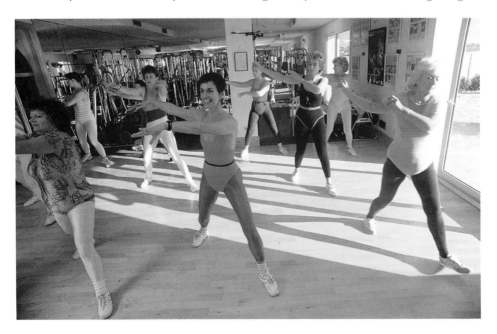

sessions of exercise at irregular intervals. It's more helpful to set aside 20 minutes every other day, than to exercise furiously for an hour every two weeks.

Yoga can be very helpful in both aiding relaxation and improving muscle tone which aids the digestive system in working more smoothly and effectively. More vigorous exercise such as swimming or aerobics, especially when combined with stretching exercises, will also help combat constipation and generally make muscles more flexible as they become stronger.

Posture can also contribute to many digestive problems, especially when it is compounded by having a job which involves spending many hours a day hunched over a desk. Because so many of us today have jobs which are both sedentary and stressful, our digestive systems are often the first things to suffer. This makes the need for exercise even stronger, even if it only involves walking upstairs instead of automatically taking the lift, or walking around the block to do some shopping instead of taking the car.

Therapies which look specifically at postural problems can also be something to consider if you have digestive problems, especially when these are combined with lower back pain. The Alexander Technique, Yoga, Osteopathy, and Chiropractic are all worth considering as possible sources of help.

Apart from looking at your diet and general lifestyle, it's worth taking a look at the problems associated with habitual use of antacids and laxatives.

Problems associated with the daily use of antacids include the syndrome of Acid Rebound which involves a vicious circle of dilution of stomach acids, followed by the stomach pumping in more acid to rectify the situation, as a result of which more antacids are taken, and so on. Some antacids also contain aluminium, which can contribute to constipation and has been linked to the development of pre-senile dementia: others contain bicarbonate of soda, which leads to water retention, and should not be used over long periods by those suffering from kidney malfunction.

Laxatives cause their own problems when used on a long-term basis. The main problem associated with regular use of laxatives (and this applies as much to a 'natural' herbal laxative as to any other) is the tendency of the bowel to lose the capacity to empty itself without the stimulation of a laxative. Once this happens, the problem of being 'hooked' on laxatives begins; this rather resembles the vicious cycle I have described in my discussion of Acid Rebound.

To end on an optimistic note, do not get discouraged if all this seems foreign to you. Selecting the most appropriate remedy takes time, some effort, and a little bit of practice. However, once you become more familiar with the remedies it gets progressively easier and you will become more confident. But above all, once you achieve positive results you will have the encouragement to continue.

5

HOMOEOPATHY AND EMOTIONAL SYMPTOMS

Emotional problems

Short-term emotional problems such as anxiety over a specific event, or the transient depression that may follow an upsetting experience, are often seen as problems that may not require help from drugs, since they will often sort themselves out. If, on the other hand, the condition seems to be either so severe that it is incapacitating, or if it appears to be going on longer than one might reasonably expect, tranquillisers or anti-depressants may well be suggested for short-term use. The rationale behind giving these drugs is that while they cannot remove the problems faced by the patient, they may give some space and distance within which to sort the problems out. Unfortunately, there are side effects to these

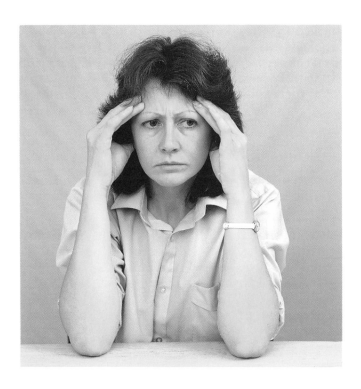

drugs which include drowsiness and fatigue, which can lead to impaired general functioning. Obviously, the long-term use of tranquillisers raises other more complex and controversial questions of physiological and psychological dependence.

Homoeopathic medicines and emotional problems

Since homoeopathic theory starts from the premise that the mind and body are inextricably interlinked, there is nothing unusual about the use of homoeopathic medicines for emotional disturbances. Because these medicines are understood to work by bringing the mind and body into an optimum state of equilibrium for the individual person, problems such as short-term anxiety need not pose an impossible problem for the prescriber. Homoeopathic medicines used appropriately in cases of short-term anxiety can be very effective in calming the person down, without involving side effects of drowsiness or fatigue. This also applies across the board to temporary sleep problems, grief or shock.

Limitations of self-prescribing for emotional problems

While it is accurate to say that homoeopathic medicines can be extremely effective in helping with emotional distress, a word of caution is needed. All of the tables in this section refer to emotional problems of recent onset in an otherwise healthy individual. If someone is suffering from long-term anxiety or depression, then it would be appropriate for that person to seek professional help from a qualified practitioner. This is needed for two reasons: Firstly, choosing an appropriate homoeopathic medicine which covers the complexity of a case of long-standing emotional problems can be a subtle business which requires experience and professional expertise. Secondly, it is important to stress that on no account does the following section suggest that the homoeopathic medicines below form substitutes for long-term use of drugs such as tranquillisers without the support of proper professional advice and treatment.

How to select the appropriate homoeopathic medicine

If you have turned to this section of the book because you are, for example, suffering from anticipatory anxiety over a coming event, this is how you would select your homoeopathic remedy.

1 Turn to the table entitled **Anticipatory Anxiety**, and look down the left hand column entitled **Type** to identify which category your symptoms fall into. If, for example, you are normally outgoing and talkative, but as the day of an exam or stressful event approaches you become increasingly withdrawn and depressed, the chances are that the column entitled 'Anticipatory anxiety with withdrawn state of mind' is likely to be most appropriate.

2 Check with the **General indications** that these symptoms fit

with your own. If you feel exhausted with worry, droopy and trembly with nerves, and are disinclined to make any physical or emotional effort, then it definitely looks like you are on the right track.

3 Finally check the **Worse from** and **Better for** columns to see if these also fit. Bear in mind that these two columns do not just refer to what makes your anxiety state better or worse, but also what might make you *generally* feel better or worse. So, if you have definitely noticed that you feel worse in a stuffy room or dwelling on the coming event, but feel much better for being occupied in the open air, the chances are that Gelsemium is the most suitable remedy for you.

4 You will find some suggestions at the end of this section of the book of general ways of minimising stress and anxiety through dietary measures, relaxation and breathing techniques.

For information on how to take the appropriate remedy, see the section entitled **How to take homoeopathic medicines** in the chapter on **Practical Homoeopathy**; exactly the same principles apply.

Anticipatory anxiety

Type	General indications	Worse from	Better for	Remedy name
Anticipatory anxiety with lots of abdominal rumbling, gurgling and wind	Anxiety often brought on by being required to speak in public. Although nervous beforehand, once begun, things go well. Anticipatory 'nerves' involve much digestive disruption: lots of wind and bloating even after only a mouthful or two of food	Being harried. When idle. Stuffy rooms	Being occupied. Open air	Lycopodium
Anticipatory anxiety with withdrawn state of mind	Exhausted, droopy and withdrawn with nervous states. Severe diarrhoea with nervous worry. Apathy with disinclination for the slightest effort. Lots of trembling and internal feelings of weakness. May feel subjectively cold	Hot room. Thinking of coming events	Open air. Stimulants. Occupation	Gelsemium

Type	General indications	Worse from	Better for	Remedy name
Anticipatory anxiety with extreme agitation and desire to engage in conversation	Fear of a coming event with feelings of panic, palpitations and tremor. Diarrhoea may be brought on by general feelings of stress and tension. Very restless with anxiety, may have a craving for sugar to keep going which aggravates the general condition	Stuffy rooms. Sweets. At night or on waking	Open air	Arg nit
Anxiety with severe vomiting, diarrhoea and restlessness	Anxiety may manifest itself in an obsessional concern with tidiness even though the person may feel exhausted. Driven by restlessness to keep going. Extreme feelings of anxiety may lead to severe involvement of the digestive system including diarrhoea and/ or vomiting. May feel extremely chilly	At night. Being alone. Cold in any form	Warmth in any form. Moving about. Company	Arsenicum album
Anxiety with dependence on stimulants to get through the event	Very irritable and overwrought with feelings of anxiety. Sleep very disturbed, often the result of needing stimulants to keep going. May suffer from constipation and general digestive irritability	Being harried. Being exposed to cold. Early morning. Stimulants	Resting undisturbed. Warmth. Napping	Nux vomica

In addition to short-term use of the appropriate homoeopathic medicine, the following suggestions may be helpful:

1 If you know that you have an event coming up which is likely to make you feel tense, try to arrange your commitments around the date so that they cause you the least amount of stress. In other words, if you know you have an exam or a driving test on a particular date, try to keep the day before it free, so that you have adequate time to prepare mentally.

2 Try to do something which you find restful on the day leading up to the event. This very much depends on you as an individual: some people might find a body massage or facial most soothing, while someone else might benefit more from a brisk walk, an exercise class or something equally vigorous.

3 If you are having problems sleeping leading up to the event, avoid stimulating drinks such as strong tea or coffee before bed, or having heavy meals before sleeping. A warm bath before bed-time using your favourite bath oil will be helpful. Generally speaking, a diet which is high in sugar, coffee, tea, or carbonated drinks is likely to make you generally more jittery before a stressful event. It's a good idea to keep them to a minimum (but don't cut them out abruptly since this can lead to withdrawal symptoms), and concentrate on soothing drinks such as chamomile tea.

4 If you notice yourself breathing quickly and from your upper chest when feeling stressed or anxious, the advice at the end of this section on breathing and relaxation will be useful to you.

Short-term insomnia

Type	General indications	Worse from	Better for	Remedy name
Sleeplessness from over-indulgence in food or alcohol	Strong mental irritability with sleeplessness. Lack of sleep may be the result of 'burning the candle at both ends'. May wake between 3–4am, then fall asleep when it's time to get up	Stimulants. Being spoken to. Cold draughts	Being left alone. Warm drinks	Nux vomica
Sleeplessness with anxiety and strong restlessness	Wakes between midnight and 2am. Very physically and mentally restless and agitated. Feels much worse if cold, and generally better for warmth. May wake with a shock after falling to sleep	Being chilled. Midnight to 2am. Being over-tired	Warmth. Warm drinks. Company	Arsenicum album
Light sleeping after grief or bad news	Violent, spasmodic yawning with inability to get a decent night's sleep. Once sleep comes it may be disturbed by bad dreams or the same repetitive nightmare. Limbs jerk on going to sleep	Emotional strain. Yawning	Change in position. Breathing deeply. Being alone	Ignatia

Type	General indications	Worse from	Better for	Remedy name
Sleeplessness from muscular over-exertion	Tosses and turns in bed trying to find a comfortable spot. The bed generally feels too hard to be comfortable. Sleeplessness may follow a day in which muscles which are unused to working are over-used. Very physically restless	Over-exertion. Being touched	Lying with head low	Arnica
Sleeplessness following a shock or disturbing experience	Panicky feelings with anxiety and restlessness. May feel convinced that they are going to die. Lots of tossing and turning, and nightmares when sleep does eventually come	Fright. In bed. Being chilled	Fresh air. Resting	Aconite
Sleeplessness from aches and pains	Great despondency with lack of ability to sleep. Aching in muscles and joints often responsible for lack of sleep. Pains may be triggered off by exposure to damp cold. Very restless with lots of tossing about and stretching	Damp and cold. Resting. After midnight	Warmth. Hot bath. Stretching.	Rhus tox
Sleeplessness with persistent drowsiness and mind which won't switch off	Irritability with sleeplessness. The mind may be occupied with work or family worries. Dreams may also reflect these preoccupations. Sleep may be disturbed by recurrent thirst, and there may generally be a difficulty in getting to sleep before midnight	Heat. Being moved. Early morning	Cool air. Cold drinks. Quiet	Bryonia

In addition to selecting the appropriate homoeopathic medicine, the following advice will be helpful:

1 Try not to continue working until bed-time, but try to do something that you find relaxing for an hour or two before you go to sleep.

2 Avoid heavy meals or stimulating drinks, such as coffee, before bed.

3 It's a good idea to have a regular pattern of exercise during the week so that your body and mind have a chance to deal with stresses and strains that naturally occur each day.

4 Have a warm bath before bed-time.

5 Try to eliminate light and noise from your room as much as possible, and make sure that it is neither too stuffy nor too cold.

6 If you cannot get to sleep, staying in bed and tossing and turning can make things worse. You could try getting up and making yourself a cup of Chamomile tea (avoiding regular tea and coffee). Once you feel sleepy enough, you could go back to bed and try again.

7 The advice at the end of this section on breathing and relaxation will also help prepare you for sleep.

8 If you suspect that your sleeplessness is becoming a long-term problem, seek professional advice rather than attempting to deal with it yourself. Insomnia would be seen by a homoeopath as a condition needing constitutional treatment (treatment which is aimed at you as a whole person with the aim of improving your overall quality of health).

Sudden grief and emotional shock

Type	General indications	Worse from	Better for	Remedy name
Fearful reaction to bad news	Often needed after witnessing an accident or being directly involved. Very frightened, restless and fearful that they may die. Lots of agitation and may seem on the verge of collapse	At night. Being touched. Noise	Rest. Open air	Aconite
Shock symptoms with desire to be left alone	Symptoms accompany physical shock: may claim that they are perfectly fine and push those who are trying to help away. May be morose mentally, but physically restless	Touch. Being approached. After sleep	Lying with head low	Arnica

Type	General indications	Worse from	Better for	Remedy name
Strong agitation and violent weeping in grief which is not resolving itself	Very helpful where someone has news of a bereavement and feels they cannot cope without help. Violent, spasmodic weeping which may alternate with bouts of laughing. Lots of twitching and tremors, with constant sighing	Touch. Cold, open air	If left alone. Eating. Breathing deeply. Near warmth	Ignatia
Grief which cannot be expressed	May want to cry, but feel they cannot in front of others, so they hold back their emotions. Consolation makes everything worse because it's likely to bring tears to the surface. Generally feels relief from being alone	Being consoled. Company. Noise	Alone. Rest. Cool air	Natrum mur
Suppressed anger from shock or bereavement	In grief may feel angry with themselves or with the person who has died for leaving them. Especially indicated where anger has been denied its natural expression. Very physically and mentally sensitive	At night. Being cold. Any sensory stimulation	Warmth. Rest	Staphysagria
Grief or shock which leads to profound tearfulness and constant need for company	Strong need for sympathy and company which helps. Very quickly moved to tears which relieve. May have a fear of being left alone	Stuffy rooms. Resting. Eating	Fresh, open air. Sympathy. After a good cry	Pulsatilla

It is worth mentioning the point that you should not feel compelled to give a homoeopathic medicine to someone who is going through their reactions to grief and coping with them. In this situation, it is perfectly normal and necessary for someone to discharge the emotions relating to their grief. If, however, they are clearly in need of extra help and support, or if the grieving process seems to be holding them back from getting on with their lives and not resolving itself, then short-term homoeopathic prescribing can be immensely helpful.

In addition to choosing the most appropriate homoeopathic medicine, the following suggestions may also be helpful:

1 Unfortunately, many bereaved people find that in the first few days and weeks following the event they are surrounded by supportive and caring friends and relations, but in the months that follow this cannot be maintained. Sadly, it often takes some months for someone to begin to accept that a death has taken place, and this is frequently the time when most support is needed but is not available. Close friends and family can be immensely important at this time in listening to how the bereaved person feels about their past and the future. This is likely to take time, but having someone to listen can help the person suffering a loss work through this phase. If it looks like the grieving person needs a more objective ear, then counselling can be very helpful in supporting them, and often leading them to insights into their emotional responses.

2 If you have experienced a shock or bereavement, try not to push yourself too hard too soon. The body and mind are likely to need space within which to recover, and this can take time. If this need is ignored, it can have the effect of leaving someone tired and exhausted for an extended period, when a shorter interval of complete rest at the appropriate time can have them back on their feet sooner.

Beyond homoeopathy: general advice

Breathing

Breathing is one of the basic functions which is essential to preserving life, and yet it is astounding how little attention most of us pay to it. Because it can be classed as an involuntary function many of us just take it for granted that we may be concentrating on something totally different, and still we continue to take oxygen in, and breathe out carbon dioxide. And yet, breathing can be the key to making us feel more or less stressed and anxious in a potentially threatening situation. I have myself experienced the strain of being asked to reverse my car on my driving test, and having accomplished the task having the examiner point out to me that it really was not necessary to stop breathing in order to accomplish the manoeuvre well! Holding one's breath or breathing rapidly and shallowly from the upper chest are two of the commonest ways of reacting to a situation which is fraught with anxiety. Unfortunately, this only makes the situation worse since the balance of oxygen and carbon dioxide in the body is disrupted, leading to more feelings of anxiety and stress which in turn cause more hyperventilation, and so the vicious circle is perpetuated.

There is however, a positive side to all of this, since if we know how to use our breathing most effectively in a crisis, it is possible to break the vicious circle outlined above, and use the breath to help us relax, feel calmer, and more in control of the situation instead of the situation controlling us.

Next time you are feeling anxious or stressed, take a moment to observe how you are breathing. The chances are that you are breathing more rapidly than usual, and that the breaths you are taking in are very shallow. Also watch what part of your chest is doing all the work, and you will probably notice that all of the effort is coming from your upper chest. In order to help yourself feel more relaxed and calm, it is necessary to learn how to breathe using your diaphragm. At first it will probably feel a little strange, but once you have got the basic idea outlined below it will improve with time and practice.

Lie on your back with your knees bent and feet on the floor. Put one hand on your belly just above your navel and watch what happens as you breathe. In order to achieve diaphragmatic breathing, as you breathe in feel the hand resting on your belly being gently pushed up, and sinking down as you breathe out. The sequence you are trying to achieve on breathing in, is first inflation of the belly followed by the chest, and on breathing out, initial flattening of the chest followed by the belly. Try not to force this process too quickly as this will probably leave you just feeling tense and frustrated, but gently and slowly take a few breaths in and out becoming conscious of the action of your diaphragm.

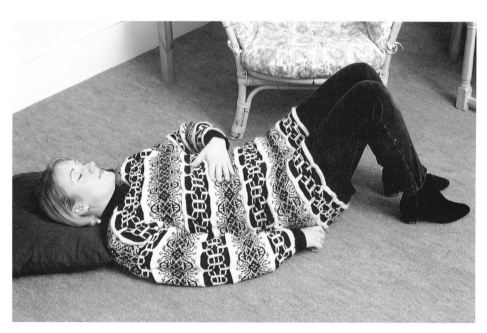

If you feel a little light-headed just stop for a while and breathe normally, you have probably been breathing too deeply or too quickly, or both. Once you feel back to normal, try again, always stopping if you need to. Once you have become familiar with this method, you can continue practising sitting upright in a chair with your hand in the same

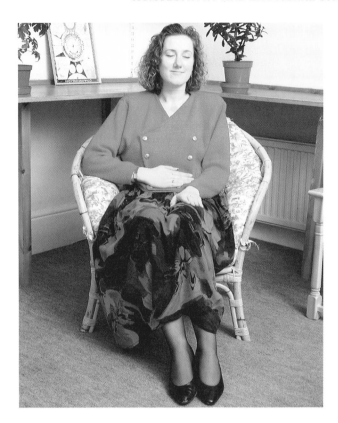

position. Try to practise breathing this way for a few minutes each day, and you will soon find that you have got the basic idea. Once it has been grasped, you can use your breathing to help you in any stressful situation.

Relaxation

When we speak of relaxation, this need not be limited to specific relaxation techniques but can embrace a range of activities from listening to music, attending an exercise class, to having a warm bath. Whatever enables you to enjoy a sensation of relaxation and well-being is very important to identify, since it will play a major role in helping you relax when you are faced with a stressful event.

Perhaps the most important point about relaxing is that this is time that you are setting aside for yourself. If you are under strain it's very easy to forget that this is the very situation where you can benefit most from time spent in this way. Ironically, it's at times like these that most of us feel that either we're too hard pushed to look after ourselves, or it's the last thing we feel like doing. Given this sort of situation, learning to value looking after yourself by taking just ten minutes or half an hour doing something that you enjoy, will leave you feeling refreshed and more able to cope. Above all, don't feel you have to fit in with other people's ideas of what constitutes a relaxing activity: find out what suits you as an individual, and most of all enjoy it.

Diet and stress

There are certain foods that should be avoided in situations of general stress and anxiety, since they can have the effect of compounding the problem. These include foods that fit in to the 'quick fix' category, in other words, foods that will stimulate you to activity in the short-term, but leave a residual feeling of exhaustion. The main offenders are coffee, strong tea, carbonated drinks including caffeine and a high sugar content, chocolate, and refined cakes and biscuits including a high proportion of sugar. If you are already feeling jittery about a coming event, and having trouble sleeping over it, depending on these foods will only kick your system into a higher state of arousal, making you feel more on edge. They also have the unfortunate effect of initially boosting your blood sugar level, which then drops dramatically, leaving you feeling tired, exhausted, and most likely irritable as well.

If you are feeling agitated and stressed, try altering the balance by cutting down on the foods mentioned above, and replacing them with foods that avoid the peaks and troughs. These include fresh and dried fruit, teas which are known to have a calming effect such as Chamomile, and as much freshly-prepared food as possible, concentrating on fish, poultry, and as many fresh vegetables as possible. Try to have a regular eating pattern, rather than going long periods of time without eating and then snatching a snack when you can.

The general idea is to try and get the broad principles right, rather than feeling you have to get everything absolutely perfect at once, since this is only likely to lead to your feeling even more under stress, and defeats the object of the exercise.

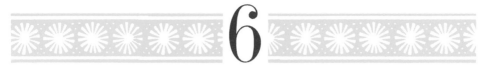

6

HOMOEOPATHY FOR CHILDHOOD ILLNESSES

Childhood infectious illnesses

Since the bulk of childhood infectious illnesses are viral in nature, there is little that the orthodox medical profession can offer as a way of dealing with the symptoms of such infections. Current measures available tend to concentrate either on ways of making the child comfortable, such painkillers, or soothing topical preparations if there is a skin eruption once the infection has set in. The other increasingly promoted and controversial method of dealing with childhood infections is the use of vaccination in the belief that it will act as a prophylactic agent, thus bypassing the susceptibility to disease. For a survey of books which deal with the complex and troubling issue of vaccination, see the Further Reading chapter at the back of this book.

Homoeopathic medicines and childhood illness

Because homoeopathic medicines are understood to work by stimulating the body's own defence mechanism to deal more effectively with disease, rather than attempting to find the specific agent which will fight the invading organism, infectious childhood illnesses pose no greater problem than any other disease to the homoeopath. Infectious illnesses are viewed by many homoeopaths as an opportunity for the young child's developing immune system to be given a 'trial run', thus helping strengthen it for the future. When the appropriate homoeopathic medicine is used to treat a child suffering from an infectious disease pain will be eased, skin eruptions often cease to be as distressing, and the general course of the disease should be speeded up. The same also applies to the non-infectious childhood problems such as teething, since homoeopathy has gained many supporters from desperate mothers who have found homoeopathic medicines to be enormously speedy and effective in dealing with the general trauma of teething.

How to select the appropriate homoeopathic medicine

If you have turned to this section of the book in order to find the appropriate homoeopathic remedy to help your child who is suffering from the early stage of measles, this is how you set about it.

1 Turn to the table entitled **Measles**, and look down the left hand column entitled **Type** to identify which category your child's symptoms fall into. If your child is normally lively and outgoing, but since being unwell is more withdrawn, tired, and apathetic, the chances are that the column entitled 'Early stage of illness with lethargy and great weariness' is likely to be most appropriate.

2 Check with the **General indications** that these symptoms fit with your child's. If he or she is achy, shivery, and looks generally droopy and heavy-lidded, then this confirms your selection. If not, try again.

3 Finally, check the **Worse from** and **Better for** columns to see if these also fit. Do bear in mind that these two columns do not just refer to what makes your child's symptoms better or worse, but also what might make him or her *generally* better or worse. So, if you have noticed that he or she feels worse for making even the slightest effort, but improves when exposed to fresh, open air, the chances are that Gelsemium will be the most helpful remedy.

4 Don't worry if **all** the symptoms mentioned in connection with Gelsemium are not present in your child; remember that what you are looking for is the closest approximation to the overall picture presented by him or her. What you do need are some major keynotes to work with, in other words, one would not give Gelsemium to a child who did not seem shivery and withdrawn, or Belladonna to a child who was not flushed and agitated.

For information on how to take the appropriate remedy, see the section entitled **How to take homoeopathic medicines** in the chapter on **Practical Homoeopathy**; exactly the same principles apply.

Measles

Type	General indications	Worse from	Better for	Remedy name
Early stage of illness with fearfulness and anxiety	Sudden onset of illness – often violent in intensity. Child is very restless and fearful, may be much worse at night. Catarrhal nasal discharge with very light-sensitive red eyes. Skin may feel burning as well as itchy. Hard sounding, croupy cough	Warm rooms. Night	Open air	Aconite

Type	General indications	Worse from	Better for	Remedy name
Early stage of illness with hot, bright red, feverish skin	Like Aconite, very swift onset of symptoms. Skin is so hot and dry that one can feel heat radiating from it. Very irritable and restless with illness. Feels drowsy but can't sleep. Throbbing head pains may accompany illness	Light. Noise. Stimulation	Lying quietly propped up in bed	Belladonna
Early stage of illness with lethargy and great weariness	Slow onset of illness with alternating high temperature, chills and shivering. Drowsy, lethargic and apathetic with drooping eyelids. Face may appear deep red and puffy. Aversion to moving even the head	Making any effort	Open air. Urinating	Gelsemium
Measles with marked distressing eye symptoms	Lots of streaming discharges from the eyes with pronounced light sensitivity. Discharge from the eyes is burning and painful, while nasal discharge is bland. Nose and eye symptoms improve from exposure to open air. Hoarseness may accompany dry cough	Light. Warmth. Evening	Open air. Blinking or wiping eye	Euphrasia
Measles with swelling of the face, eyes, and eyelids	The rash may appear slowly with characteristic stinging pains. Rosy pink, puffy, and itching eruptions which are relieved by cool bathing	Heat. Touch. After sleep	Cool air and cool bathing	Apis
Later stage of measles, once the rash has come out and fever has subsided	Dry mouth with no thirst. Cough alternates between dry at night and loose in the morning. Catarrh is bland, thick and yellow-green in colour. Rash feels worse for warmth and better for cool air. Ear pain may develop. Weepy with symptoms	Stuffy rooms. Rest. Warmth. Eating	Cool, open air. Gentle motion	Pulsatilla

Type	General indications	Worse from	Better for	Remedy name
Measles with rash slow to develop with marked chest symptoms	Chesty cough causing pain in chest. Lots of tickling and irritation in larynx. Headache accompanies cough and feels much worse for motion. Dry mouth with intense thirst for cold drinks. May be constipated and generally irritable with symptoms	Least motion. Sitting up. Becoming heated. Eating	Cool, open air. Quiet. Cold drinks	Bryonia

The following advice will be supportive of homoeopathic treatment.

1 Encourage the child to drink as much fluid as possible. If he or she has a high temperature, they are unlikely to be hungry and it will not help to force food on them at this stage, but plenty of liquid is essential.

2 If there is light sensitivity, ensure that light is kept to a minimum by dimming lights, or drawing curtains.

If any of the following occur, prompt professional help is advised:

1 Breathing difficulties.

2 Temperature registering over 104°.

3 If your child is under six months of age.

4 Earache.

5 Severe headache, lethargy, drowsiness or vomiting.

6 Bleeding from orifices or under the skin.

7 If cough is persistent for more than four days.

8 Any sign of eye infection.

9 If the temperature doesn't resolve itself as the rash develops.

Mumps

Type	General indications	Worse from	Better for	Remedy name
Rapid onset of mumps symptoms with terrific heat and redness	Marked restlessness with high temperature. Glands adjacent to the ears may look red and feel tender to touch. The right side may be particularly affected. Dry, burning throat with thirstlessness. Shooting pains in glands ands throbbing headache	Touch. Light. Noise	Lying down	Belladonna
Mumps with sensation of pressure and tension in glands	Hard, tense stony feelings in glands adjacent to the ear lobe and under the jaw. Dry throat with difficulty swallowing, pains shoot to the ears when attempting to swallow. Face and skin in general look pale (the opposite of Belladonna)	At night. Cold and damp. Warmth of bed. Swallowing warm food or drink	Warmth in general	Phytolacca
Mumps with copious salivation and marked weakness	Marked sweat is followed by profuse perspiration. Dry mouth with free salivation, and marked dryness at the back of the throat. Tonsils may be swollen and jaws are likely to feel stiff. Speech may be difficult with coating of the tongue	Cold		Jaborandi
Mumps with offensive breath and copious salivation and sweat	Sweating much worse with onset of night. Unpleasant sweet, metallic taste in the mouth with bad breath and swollen tongue. Most likely to be indicated in the later stages of the illness, once the fever has peaked	Night. Extreme temperature changes. Draught. Sweat	Rest	Merc sol

Type	General indications	Worse from	Better for	Remedy name
Mumps with marked rosy, red swellings and heat sensitivity	Pains are stinging and feel much better for cool applications. Swellings are pronounced and look very puffy. Eyelids may look especially swollen. Constantly fidgety and restless	Warmth. Lying down. After sleep	Cool air. Cool applications. Change of position	Apis
Mumps with marked irritability and sensitivity to movement	Extreme sensitivity to motion, even of single limbs. Lethargic and wants to be left alone to lie still. Slow, insidious onset of illness with possible involvement of stubborn constipation. Marked thirst for large quantities of cold drinks with dry lips	Moving. Heat. Effort	Lying still. Perspiration	Bryonia
Mumps with pain which is much worse on the left side	Extreme sensitivity and swelling of the glands on the left side. Marked aversion to touch or pressure. Throbbing and constrictive pains. Swallowing is extremely painful and difficult	After sleep. Touch. Empty swallowing. Tight clothes around the neck	Open air. Cold drinks. Eating	Lachesis
Lingering mumps with involvement of breasts or testes in adults	Symptoms feel generally worse for heat and better for open air. Child may be whiny, clingy, and generally attention-seeking. Dry mouth with coated tongue and lack of thirst	Stuffy rooms. Lying down. At night	Open air. Gentle movement. Consolation	Pulsatilla
Mumps symptoms which feel much worse for exposure to damp cold, and are much worse at night	Marked swelling of glands which may be much worse on the left than the right. Extreme restlessness and despondency at night with terrific sensitivity to cold and chilliness. May have cold sores on the lips. Dreadful aching in the limbs which rest aggravates	Cold and damp. At night. Rest	Heat. Warm bathing. Being wrapped up warmly	Rhus tox

1 It is helpful to withhold acid drinks and spicy food from children when they have mumps since they will stimulate salivation which will lead to increased pain.

2 Avoid children who are suffering from mumps being in contact with adults who have not contracted the disease, since the complications in adults can be very unpleasant. These include painful swelling of the testicles in males, and inflammation of the ovaries and/or the breasts in women.

If any of the following occur you should consider seeking professional advice:

1 Stiff neck accompanied by weakness and/or headache or convulsions.

2 Inflammation of the breasts or testes in adults who have been in contact with the disease.

3 Difficulties with hearing or vision.

4 Abdominal pains, especially if accompanied by vomiting.

Chicken-pox

Type	General indications	Worse from	Better for	Remedy name
Chicken-pox with very itchy rash and extreme restlessness which is much worse at night	Dreadful itching which is made worse by scratching. Everything feels much worse at night, and there is likely to be much difficulty getting to sleep. Very chilly and cold sensitive	Scratching. At night. Cold	Warm bathing. Moderate temperature	Rhus tox
Chicken-pox where the rash is very slow to develop	Large, slow to develop rash with accompanying rattling cough. Very bad tempered with symptoms, tendencies to moan and whine. Skin may be cold with a blue or pustular rash. Tongue may be white and thickly-coated	Cold. Lying down	Cool air. Bringing up phlegm	Ant tart
Chicken-pox with flushed, hot, red skin and raised temperature	Very hot, bright red skin which feels very dry to the touch. Lots of drowsiness with inability to sleep. Throbbing headache with tendency to be sensitive to slightest stimulation	Noise. Bright light	Rest. Warm room	Belladonna

Type	General indications	Worse from	Better for	Remedy name
Chicken-pox with marked desire for warmth	Chilly, restless and anxious. Eruptions look large and contain lots of pus. All symptoms generally seem worse at night	At night. Effort. Cold	Warmth. Lying with head raised	Arsenicum album
Chicken-pox with swollen glands and offensive, copious sweat	Reacts badly to either strong heat or cold, and at night. Large eruptions with a lot of pus that may develop into sores. Sweat and breath are likely to be profuse and offensive. May complain of metallic taste in the mouth and increased salivation	Heat. Cold. At night	Resting	Merc sol
Chicken-pox with low grade fever and weepiness	Likely to be the later stages of chicken-pox with swollen glands and lingering low-grade temperature. Child feels weepy and clingy and demands attention. Complains of chilliness, but feels better for open air	Stuffy rooms. At night. Resting. Warmth	Open air. Gentle motion. Cool	Pulsatilla

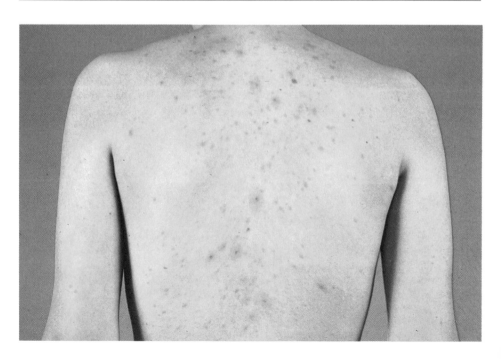

The following measures are generally helpful in easing symptoms:

1 Try ways of preventing your child from scratching the eruptions since this can lead to infection and scarring. One way of avoiding this is to trim the fingernails fairly short.

2 After bathing don't rub at the eruptions, but try to pat them dry gently to avoid damaging the scabs.

3 If the skin is very itchy an oatmeal bath may be soothing, or try applying a diluted solution of Urtica urens tincture to the itchy areas of skin (available from homoeopathic pharmacies).

4 If your child is not hungry don't feel compelled to push food on him or her. Meals should be kept as light and as easily digestible as possible.

5 Avoid using aspirin since it may be implicated in the development of Reye's Syndrome (a serious illness characterised by high temperature, vomiting and problems with liver and kidneys).

If any of the following occur, professional help should be seriously considered:

1 Severe headache, marked weakness, convulsions or stiff neck.

2 Vomiting or rapid, shallow respiration.

3 Bleeding under the skin.

4 Infection of skin eruption.

5 Chicken-pox in a child of less than one year of age.

Whooping cough

Type	General indications	Worse from	Better for	Remedy name
Whooping cough with clammy, cold sweat	In bouts of coughing the child turns initially red and then becomes pale, cold and clammy. Strong desire for cool, fresh air. Burning sensations in chest with the rawness of larynx and trachea. Cough is initially hard and dry, but lots of mucus is produced after the cough	At night. Warmth. Walking	Cool air. Fanning	Carbo veg

Type	General indications	Worse from	Better for	Remedy name
Whooping cough with wheezing, rattling cough	Child stiffens in a coughing bout and loses breath. Skin may take on a bluish shade in a coughing spasm. Episode of coughing ends in gagging and vomiting. Nosebleeds may accompany the cough	Damp air. Lying. Motion	Open air. Rest. Cold drinks	Ipecac
Dry, metallic-sounding whooping cough with hoarseness	Severe bouts of coughing which follow each other in quick succession. Barking cough comes from deep in abdomen. The cough generally starts as soon as the child lies down	At night. Resting. Talking. Warmth	In open air. Being active	Drosera
Whooping cough which is worse in stuffy rooms	Episodes of coughing provoked by trying to clear throat of mucus. Coughing ends with vomiting of stringy mucus which hangs from the mouth	Stuffy rooms. Warmth	Sips of water	Coccus cacti
Whooping cough with sensations of smothering preceding bouts of coughing	Profuse nasal catarrh may accompany the cough, but the cough is likely to be dry. After coughing, vomiting of stringy mucus. Feels too cold when uncovered, and too hot when covered	Change of air. Inhaling air. Eating	Heat	Corallium rubrum
Whooping cough with easy expectoration	Chest feels sensitive during coughing bout. Dry, barking cough in cold air, becoming very loose once in warm room. Choking sensation followed by vomiting	Cold. Draught. Being heated. After exertion	Open air. Moderate warmth	Kali carb
Whooping cough with sore and bruised feelings in the chest	Cough aggravated during sleep and on exercise. Child may cry before cough sets in anticipating the pain. Because of bruised feelings, child may hold the chest when coughing	Damp cold. Exertion	Resting	Arnica

See the general advice in the Cough section of the chapter on the Respiratory System. In addition the following measures may be helpful:

1 Reassurance by a parent can do a lot to alleviate panic accompanying coughing bouts.

2 Small meals and drinks are best given just after a coughing bout.

3 Young babies can be assisted when coughing by holding them face down, while older children are helped by leaning forward while sitting.

4 Guard against dehydration by keeping fluid intake adequate.

For advice on when to seek help, turn to the Cough section, bearing in mind that special attention needs to be given to small babies since they are more vulnerable to complications.

Earache

Type	General indications	Worse from	Better for	Remedy name
Rapid onset of pain after exposure to dry, cold winds	Lots of anxiety and hypersensitivity to pain. Temperature may be high, with accompanying thirst and congested appearance. Noise causes great distress. Very restless	Noise. Warm rooms. At night	Sleep. Open air	Aconite
Violent, sudden onset, with very high temperature and redness	Tendency for the pain to lodge in the right side. Pains are violent, throbbing, and burning. Lots of irritability with the pains. Ear pain may extend to the neck with accompanying sore throat and facial pain	Stimulation. Being touched. Moving	Lying still. Heat	Belladonna
Early stage of earache which is milder than the indications for Aconite or Belladonna	May be either flushed or pale with pain, or alternate between the two. Early stages of earache where pus has not yet formed. Itching sensations in the ear with drawing pains	Open air. Exertion. Noise	Gentle motion	Ferrum phos

Type	General indications	Worse from	Better for	Remedy name
Earache with extreme irritability and screaming.	The pain puts the child in an extremely bad temper. Refuses to be comforted, but may be soothed by being carried. Pains feel worse for bending over. May repeatedly try to cover ear for relief of pain	Cold air. Bending over	Warmth. Being carried. Being wrapped up	Chamomilla
Earache that accompanies the established stage of a cold	Nasal discharge which is bland, thick, and yellow-green in colour. Earache may be severe, or cause little distress in the child. May feel chilly, but reacts badly to warm rooms. Child may be uncharacteristically weepy or clingy	Stuffy rooms. Warmth. At night. Rest	Cool. Gentle motion	Pulsatilla
Earache which accompanies the middle stage of a cold, with thin discharge from the ear	Lots of weariness with cold and earache. Feels chilly and generally better for being warmly wrapped up. Itching in the ear or stuffed-up feeling	At night. Cold applications. Moving. Lying on painful side	Warmth. Being well wrapped up	Silica
Earache with extreme cold sensitivity and irritability	Discharges are thick and coloured. Cold makes the child very uncomfortable and bad-tempered, while wrapping up warm tends to be soothing. Pains are sticking and bursting	At night. Cold draught	Heat. Being covered up snuggly	Hepar sulph
Earache with offensive, profuse sweating and discharges	Reacts very badly to extremes of temperature and to being in bed at night. Lots of salivation with possible metallic taste in mouth and flabby tongue. May also have glandular involvement	Cold or heat. In bed. Sweating	Moderate tempera-tures	Merc sol

The following measures will be helpful in minimising pain and discomfort, and speeding up the healing process:

1 Drinking plenty of liquids will help flush toxins out of the body. Be careful to avoid milk and milk products since these are thought to contribute to mucus formation.

2 As with any other infectious illness, it is very important to rest in order to allow the body to recover as quickly as possible.

3 A warm flannel or heating pad could be applied to the ear if the pain responds well to heat.

If any of the following occur, professional help should be strongly considered:

1 If there is any weakness, lethargy, stiff neck or severe headache.

2 If a baby is pulling or rubbing its ear.

3 Any discharge in a child under the age of seven.

4 Any redness or tenderness in the bony area behind the ear.

5 Any sudden or noticeable decrease in hearing with or without pain.

6 If discharge lasts in an older child longer than one or two weeks.

7 If hearing loss persists for more than two weeks.

Croup

Type	General indications	Worse from	Better for	Remedy name
Croup with extreme anxiety and restlessness	Early on in the bout of croup with high temperature and restlessness. Cough is very dry, loud and barking. The larynx may be sensitive to touch, and the child may grasp at the throat. Croup may follow soon after exposure to dry, cold air	Cold air. At night. Breathing in. Touch. Warm room	Open air. Sweating	Aconite
Croup with distinctive sound as though a saw was being drawn through dry wood	Wheezing and rasping with croup with difficulty breathing between spasms. Cough sounds raw and dry with accompanying sense of suffocation. If indicated, it follows Aconite well. Not as anxious with fever as Aconite	Swallowing. Exertion. Talking. Heat	Warm food. Warm drinks. Lying with head low	Spongia

Type	General indications	Worse from	Better for	Remedy name
Croup with extreme cold sensitivity and irritability	Rattling cough with suffocative spells. Hoarse and wheezy with difficulty in breathing. Very mentally and physically touchy and dissatisfied	Early morning. Cold air. Draught	Moist heat. After eating. Warm wraps to head	Hepar sulph
Croup which has passed the violent stage of recent onset, but keeps relapsing	Hoarseness and complete loss of voice may accompany croup. Tickly, dry cough which responds temporarily to cold drinks. Lots of anxiety and restlessness accompany croup, with a strong desire for sympathy and attention	At night. Cold air. Touch	Sleep. Eating. Cold food and water until they become warm in stomach	Phosphorus
Croup with metallic sounding, brassy, hacking cough	Cough with thick yellow mucus discharged from the mouth and nose. Troublesome tickling in larynx with cough. Dry, burning, raw sensation in the throat. Hoarse voice worse in the evening. Generally indifferent with aversion to the slightest exertion	Morning. Evening. Cold and damp	Heat. Motion. Bringing up phlegm. Pressure	Kali bich

Keeping fluid intake up and putting the child in a steam filled bathroom will both help ease the condition. Reassurance is also needed for the child, since croup can be a very distressing experience.

If the child shows marked difficulty in breathing accompanied by drooling from the mouth, or you are in the least bit unsure about the seriousness of the condition, do seek professional help promptly.

Teething

Type	General indications	Worse from	Better for	Remedy name
Teething which leads to terrific temper and screaming	Baby constantly puts fingers in mouth seeking for relief. Pain causes screaming and extreme irritability which nothing seems to comfort. May get to the point of screaming and hitting out at those around. May only respond to being carried constantly	At night. Heat. Open air	Being rocked or carried	Chamomilla
Teething which causes great distress and weeping	More weepy than irritable with teething. Sighing, sobbing and jerking may accompany teething symptoms. May be woken from sleep with piercing cries of distress	After drinking	Biting. Pressure	Ignatia
Teething with high temperature and extreme pain sensitivity	Baby is flushed, hot and dry-skinned. Very sensitive to any sensual stimulation. Cheeks look red, hot and swollen. Very drowsy, but sleep is restless	Noise. Touch. Jarring	Lying semi-propped up in bed	Belladonna
Teething with whining and need for sympathy	Pains may be tearing and stitching making the child weepy and needing a lot of affection	Stuffy rooms. Warm drinks	Cool, open air. Cool drinks	Pulsatilla
Teething with severe inflammation of the gums	Spongy, inflamed gums which look very red. Child is likely to behave in a very agitated way when teething. Wakeful at night. Earache may accompany teething pains	Cold. At rest. Lying down	Warm. Movement	Kreosotum

Type	General indications	Worse from	Better for	Remedy name
Teething with slow emergence of teeth, and diarrhoea	Very painful and slow teething. Colds and coughs may accompany teething process as well as green-coloured diarrhoea. Closure of fontanelles may be delayed	Damp and cold	Warm and dry	Calc phos

Using a teething toy filled with cold water, or a flannel wrapped around some ice for your child to bite on, may do a lot to ease discomfort. Generally speaking, the most soothing things to gnaw on are soft, cool, and firm.

Colic

Type	General indications	Worse from	Better for	Remedy name
Colic which is relieved by pressure	Colic leads to baby doubling up and screaming with pain. Generally restless, irritable and angry. Pain in abdomen also feels better for warm applications. May have coated tongue	At rest. Motion. Eating. Drinking	Bending double. Firm pressure. Lying on stomach. Passing wind	Colocynthis
Colic with violent temper and screaming relieved by being nursed	Moans and screams with pain. Very irritable, restless and hard to please. May have accompanying diarrhoea which is green and offensive. Looks distended after eating	Burping	Heat. Being carried	Chamomilla
Colic which responds very well to warm applications	Very sensitive to cold draughts and generally anxious with pain. Lots of bloating with wind leading to restless behaviour. Clean tongue with colicky pains	At night. Cold. Being stretched out. Motion	Doubling up. Warmth. Rubbing. Belches	Mag phos

Type	General indications	Worse from	Better for	Remedy name
Colic which is much worse for movement	Very irritable and cross. The baby doesn't seem to know what it wants. May have constipation with colic and a marked thirst for cold drinks. Pains generally worse for warm applications	Moving. Warmth. Eating	Rest. Firm pressure	Bryonia

Always seek professional advice if any of the following occur with baby colic:

1 Any signs of dehydration: Sunken fontanelles (soft spot at the crown of the head); sunken eyes; strong or decreased amount of urine passed; dry mouth or eyes; loss of skin tone.

2 If pain in the abdomen appears to be severe.

3 Vomiting and diarrhoea accompanying colicky pain, or constipation.

4 Lethargy, screaming or changed behaviour with colicky pain.

Beyond homoeopathy: general advice

In conclusion, it is worth mentioning that one should never be in doubt about calling on professional help if worried about a child's condition. Without being alarmist, it is worth bearing in mind that potentially serious childhood illnesses can develop rapidly and need identifying as quickly as possible. Unlike adults, children can get dramatically sick very quickly, so if there is any doubt in your mind, do get advice.

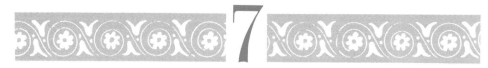

7

QUESTIONS AND ANSWERS ABOUT HOMOEOPATHIC TREATMENT

How can I find a homoeopathic practitioner?

The Society of Homoeopaths will supply a register of qualified professional homoeopaths who have undergone a minimum of four years training at an approved homoeopathic college. If you require a list of orthodox doctors who also practise homoeopathy you should contact The British Homoeopathic Association.

While registers are useful in giving basic information about homoeopathic practitioners in your area, I would strongly advise you to find out if anyone you know has had successful homoeopathic treatment, since referral tends to be one of the most reliable ways of finding a reputable homoeopathic practitioner. Obviously, this may not be a foolproof method since the relationship with your homoeopath will always be unique, and what is appropriate for one person may not be so successful for another. Nevertheless, if you have heard from a friend that the homoeopath they visited was professional, knowledgeable, sensitive and perceptive to their individual needs, it would be well worth following this up with an enquiry.

This method also helps overcome the problem that there are homoeopathic practitioners who trained before the college system began, and as a result may not be included on the available registers. It also bypasses the prejudice that some people may unwittingly have towards non-doctor homoeopaths, thinking that in order to have a responsible and well-qualified homoeopath they must look for someone who has had an orthodox medical training. In reality, things are not this straightforward, since one may find excellent homoeopaths who have also trained in conventional medicine, or those have had the same orthodox medical training who view homoeopathy as nothing more than

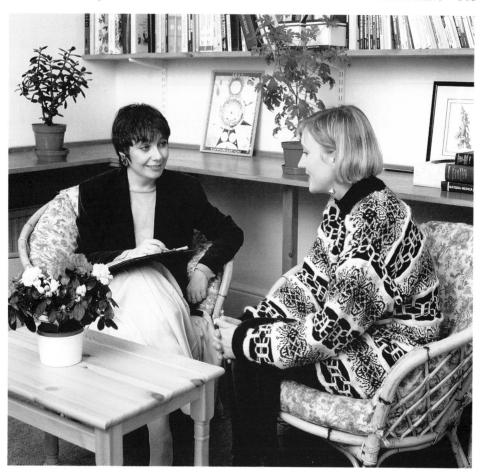

a tool of very limited usefulness due to their having received a brief and perfunctory training in it. Unfortunately in the latter situation the homoeopathic treatment received may be disappointing or misleading to the patient. It is also fair to say that there are also professional homoeopaths who may practise in an unsatisfactory way for the patient, and that this is something that cannot be conveyed by a register. As you can see, obtaining a recommendation from someone you know and whose opinion you trust will help you feel more confident about your choice of practitioner.

Should I avoid orthodox drugs if I am taking homoeopathic medicines?

Since homoeopathic medicines are understood to work on the energy levels of the sick person they leave no traceable chemical constitutents in the blood stream or tissues. As a result, they are working on an entirely different level to orthodox drugs which leave detectable traces in the body. Because of this major difference in approach and effect, there is little chance of the two medicines having an adverse interaction with each other and giving rise to undesirable side effects.

Orthodox drugs which have a strong suppressive action such as antibiotics can interrupt the action of the homoeopathic medicine, and patients who have had long courses of suppressive therapy may find that their systems take longer to respond to homoeopathic treatment. As a result, viewed in this light, we can see that there is a basic incompatibility between orthodox and homoeopathic medicines, which rests more on the level of the philosophy of illness than adverse biochemical interaction.

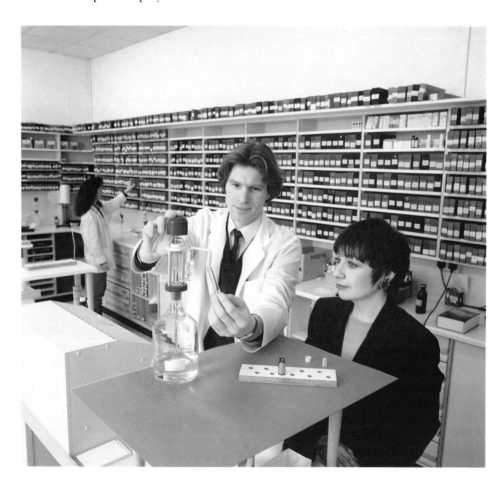

Are there certain foods I should avoid when taking homoeopathic medicines?

Some foodstuffs are thought to possibly interfere with the action of homoeopathic medicines: these include coffee, strong tea, and some herbal infusions such as peppermint (this also includes strong peppermint or spearmint-flavoured toothpaste). Always try to avoid taking a homoeopathic remedy immediately after eating or drinking when there may be strong residual flavours in the mouth.

Can homoeopathy help my sick pet?

Pets can benefit enormously from homoeopathy for the whole range of conditions affecting large and small animals alike. To obtain homoeopathic treatment for your pet, you need to contact the British Homoeopathic Association who can provide you with a list of orthodoxly-trained vets who have undergone an additional training in homoeopathy. If you do not have a homoeopathic vet in your area, enquire whether any of the vets on the list provide a telephone consultation service for routine conditions. There are a number of self-help manuals on the market for homoeopathic treatment of acute conditions in animals, which can be helpful for obvious complaints, but as always, contact a professional if you suspect you are getting out of your depth.

Do homoeopathic medicines lead to side effects?

Because homoeopathic medicines work by stimulating the body's own curative potential by boosting vital energy, side effects produced by the medicines are not a problem since there cannot be a build-up in the body. If the body is overstimulated by too frequent a repetition of a remedy, the original symptom for which the remedy was taken might get briefly worse. If this happens, all one has to do is to stop taking the remedy and, within a short space of time, things should return to where they were before the aggravation set in.

If you take a remedy that is inappropriate for a relatively short space of time (up to three doses, one hour apart) all that is likely to happen is the disappointment of no response for the better. In this situation no harm has been done, just take another detailed look at the symptoms and see if another remedy is more strongly indicated.

Always remember that the most important thing to avoid is over-frequent administration of a homoeopathic medicine. If it is working, always stop and wait. This is an indication that the body has been stimulated into action in a beneficial direction, and that it can cope very well by itself until the symptoms return. Once things start to slip back you may repeat the remedy until improvement sets in again. If it looks like a remedy has stopped having a beneficial effect, take another look at the symptoms and see if another remedy is not more strongly indicated. If not, at this stage you may consider whether a stronger dose of the original remedy is called for.

Are there situations where homoeopathy might not be of use?

Generally speaking, homoeopathic prescribing is useful in any of the self-help situations outlined in this book. Categories of problems where homoeopathic prescribing would be likely to produce disappointing results might include any situation where permanent tissue damage has occurred, problems which relate to a mechanical obstacle to recovery as in the case of displaced vertebrae, or cases where so much strong orthodox medication has been taken, that it is difficult to differentiate between the patient's original symptoms and the side effects of drug therapy.

Even in some of the situations outlined above, it is worth bearing in mind that homoeopathic prescribing may still be very helpful in minimising pain and distress as a useful adjunct to other therapies.

Can homoeopathic medicines replace antibiotics?

There is no reason why homoeopathic medicines cannot be prescribed in cases of bacterial infections with effective results, provided the prescribing is accurate and competent. As I stated earlier in this book, homoeopathic medicines are capable of aiding the body in its fight against the range of bacterial or viral infections by stimulating the body's own defence mechanism. Clearly, the results obtained will depend very much on the experience and skill of the prescriber, but it is very helpful to use the indicated homoeopathic remedy as the first resort, keeping the antibiotic in reserve if the expected improvement is not forthcoming.

It is obvious that a professional practitioner is more likely to be able to prescribe with the accuracy needed to institute a healing response in the minimum amount of time. It is also true that if a homoeopathic practitioner is professional in their approach to clinical signs and symptoms, that they will pick up indications that suggest that improvement is not forthcoming and that the situation is worsening. It must be said that effective homoeopathic treatment in skilled hands can avoid the over-use of antibiotics, leaving the latter as a last ditch strategy for those situations which are sluggish in response to more holistic measures.

As always, never proceed with self-help prescribing if you feel the situation is deteriorating and you are feeling anxious about it. Do get professional help and advice rather than feeling you must soldier on by yourself.

Should I have my child vaccinated if he or she is receiving homoeopathic treatment?

The issue of vaccination is one that is fraught with controversy because of the emotive nature of the debate with regard to children. Many homoeopaths will present a strong argument against immunisation, arguing that vaccines do not provide long-term immunity to the diseases being vaccinated for, and that there may be long-term side effects following vaccination including susceptibility to recurrent ear infections, allergic reactions, and skin problems. Homoeopaths also draw attention to the different processes involved in acquiring a natural immunity to infectious disease when compared with the immune response engendered by vaccination. Infection of one child from another who has a childhood disease such as measles involves a systematic response in the infected child over an extended period of time; by the stage the symptoms of high temperature, aching and rash have appeared the immune system has begun to produce antibodies against the virus. Injection of a vaccine into the bloodstream provokes only an antibody response rather than mobilising a systemic inflammatory reaction, and may leave residual viral elements of the body for an extended period of time.

Clearly, the whole issue of vaccinating, or not vaccinating your child is one that can be fraught with guilt, confusion, and anxiety. If you consult a homoeopath about yourself or your child, I would suggest you discuss the issue with them in detail, especially with regard to what homoeopathic measures can be taken in the situation of a child developing one of the infectious childhood illnesses. There is also a growing number of books and articles available on this subject which I would suggest you read before making an informed decision either way. The material included in these publications should make it easier for you to have a useful discussion with your family doctor or your health visitor about this very complex issue. If you would like more information on this subject turn to the Further Reading chapter.

Can I use other alternative therapies if I am receiving homoeopathic treatment?

Most therapies that fall into the 'alternative' category, such as massage, osteopathy, chiropactic, reflexology, or autogenic training, can be used side by side with homoeopathy. Any therapy which has at its heart the aim of helping the individual achieve the maximum amount of balance and harmony in mind and body, has a very similar aim to homoeopathy as a system of healing. Yoga and the Alexander Technique may both be helpful in teaching the homoeopathic patient more about the way they move and respond to stress, while basic relaxation techniques can do a great deal to help someone come to terms with how they deal with the amount of mental and emotional strain they may have in their lives. Some homoeopaths suggest that acupuncture, although it has much in common with homoeopathy as a holistic system of medicine, may not work easily in harmony with homoeopathic treatment. In these cases, it is often suggested that the patient concentrates on one of these two therapies for a set period of time to assess the benefits of each independently.

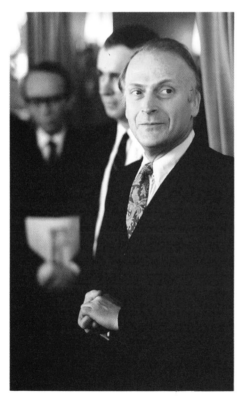

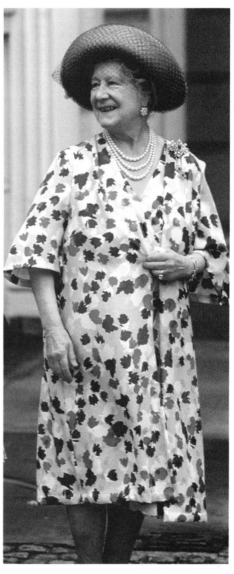

Once you begin to experience homoeopathy as a system of healing for yourself and others, it is often noticeable that a natural examination of lifestyle and diet begins. This is a very positive development, since there is little point in substituting homoeopathic medicines for orthodox drugs, if there is a underlying dietary factor which is leading to the problem as in the case of excess drinking, or a highly-indigestible diet. This most emphatically does not mean that you need to become a strict vegetarian, or give up alcohol or other foods that give pleasure in moderation: a harsh or puritan approach will not lead to a sense of balance either. But as you become more familiar with what leads your body to experience a sense of enhanced well-being and what does the reverse, the chances are that you will want to maximise your optimum level of good health by supporting your body, rather than fighting against it.

APPENDIX

Remedy keynotes

Aconite

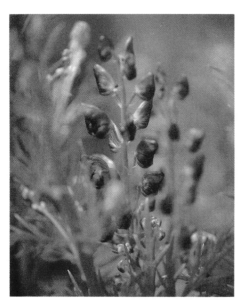

- Conditions of sudden, violent onset.
- Most likely to be of use in the first stages of illness rather than established stages.
- Very anxious with specific fear of death.
- Conditions often follow from exposure to dry, cold winds.
- Strong intolerance of pain with extreme restlessness and anxiety.
- Strong affinity for organs of respiration.

Worse from:
Night.
Warm rooms.

Better for:
Open air.

Apis

- Red, puffy swellings that appear with rapidity.
- Puffy swellings may appear around the eyes, mouth, or in the throat.
- Often indicated in allergic skin reactions.
- Stinging, burning pains that are relieved by cold.
- Conditions may follow a rash that has disappeared or failed to appear.
- Scanty urination and discharges.

Worse from:
Heat.

Better for:
Cold air and applications.

Arnica

- Indicated in the first stage of trauma, shock and bruising following accidents.

- Bruised and aching sensations with extreme restlessness.

- Weary, sore and prostrated.

- Cannot get comfortable in any position, especially in bed.

- Strong aversion to being touched; may fear the approach of anyone.

- Claim that they do not need attention, all they want is to be left alone.

Worse from:
Touch.
Heat.
Rest.

Better for:
Lying with head low.

Arsenicum album

- Pains which are generally burning: throat, stomach, skin etc.

- Acrid, burning, scanty discharches.

- Chilly and prostrated by illness.

- Marked anxiety and restlessness which is aggravated at night.

- Strong affinity for organs of digestion and respiration.

- Wants air but is sensitive to cold in general.

- Peculiar symptom of burning pains relieved by warmth.

- Most symptoms are relieved by keeping warm, except for head symptoms which feel better for cool air.

Worse from:
Night, especially after midnight.
Cold (except for head).
Sight or smell of food.
Being alone.

Better for:
Warmth.
Sips of hot drinks.
Lying propped up in bed.

Belladonna

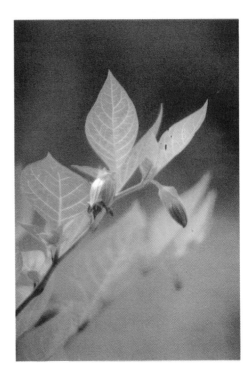

- Early stage of illness with sudden, violent onset.

- Bright red, dry skin with bounding pulse.

- Very sensitive to external impressions: light and noise, etc.

- Very agitated and irritable.

- May be delirious with dilated pupils.

- Symptoms show an affinity for the right side: earache, sore throat, etc.

- Restless sleep with muscular twitching.

Worse from:
Noise.
Light.
Lying down.
Moving.

Better for:
Sitting up in bed in a darkened room.
Keeping still in a warm room.

Bryonia

- Slow developing symptoms.

- Dryness of mucus membranes, stool, cough, etc.

- Headache may accompany most ailments.

- Irritable and touchy with illness: just want to be left alone.

- Moving makes most symptoms worse.

- Instinctive desire to press the affected part in order to hold it still, especially the chest and the head.

- Strong aversion to warmth and a general desire for cool.

- Thirst is very marked for large quantities of cold water.

Worse from:
Movement.

Heat.
After eating.

Better for:
Cold.
Keeping still.
Pressure.

Carbo veg

- Air hunger with collapse.

- Skin is pale, clammy, and tinged with blue.

- Chilly in general, but wants to be uncovered when feeling cold.

- Internal burning with external coldness.

- Lots of flatulence with heavy sensations in stomach.

Worse from:
Warmth.
Lying down.
Fatty food.

Better for:
Being fanned.
Belching.

Gelsemium

- Complaints which develop slowly over a period of days.

- Aching, weary, and exhausted sensations.

- Shivers run up and down spine.

- Everything feels heavy especially the eyelids which look droopy.

- Indifference to anything due to lack of energy.

- Congestive sensations, especially in the head.

- Dark red, deeply flushed face.

- Lethargic, incoherent, and forgetful.

- Very chilly with cold extremities.

Worse from:
Exertion.
Lying with head low.

Better for:
Bending forwards.
Open air.
Sitting still propped up by pillows.

Hepar sulph

- Very sensitive to cold and drafts of cold air.

- Peculiar and characteristic sensation of a sticking pain in the throat as though a fish bone was lodged there.

- Marked irritability, chilliness, and hypersensitivity.

- Pains are very severe, sharp and sticking.

- Lots of catarrh and a tendency to suppuration.

- Thick, yellow, offensive-smelling discharges.

- Night sweats which give no relief.

Worse from:
Cold.
Touch.
Exertion.

Better for:
Wet weather.

Warmth.
Wrapping up warmly.

Hypericum

- Marked affinity for injury to areas rich in nerve supply, e.g. fingers, toes, base of spine.

- Often indicated in puncture wounds with shooting pains.

- Use for residual nerve pain following dental work.

- Promotes healing of jagged lacerations.

Worse from:
Touch.
Cold.

Better for:
Bending head back.

Ignatia

- Muscular spasms especially affecting the digestive tract giving rise to hiccoughing.

- Repeated sighing.

- Uncontrollable weeping.

- Contradictory symptoms, e.g. indigestion relieved by eating.

- The main remedy to think of in cases of emotional shock and grief.

- Unpredictability of moods: moves quickly from one extreme to another.

Worse from:
Emotional strain.
Strong odours.
Tobacco, coffee and alcohol.

Better for:
Warmth.
Distraction.
Eating.

Lachesis

- Affinity for the throat, and left-sided complaints.

- Disturbances of the circulation, leading to a bluish-purple tinge to the skin.

- All symptoms are much worse from sleep.

- Nerves and the senses in general are likely to be overwrought.

- Throat is very sensitive to touch.

- Strong suffocative sensations: must rush for air.

- Tendency to glandular swelling and sensitivity of the neck.

Worse from:
Sleep.
Touch.
Becoming warm.

Better for:
Onset of discharge.
Fresh air.
Removing any constricting garment from around the neck.

Ledum

- Affinity for puncture wounds.

- Tendency for affected part to feel cold to the touch.

- Affected area looks red and swollen.

- Pains are throbbing.

- Strong affinity for injured joints, fibrous tissue, and tendons.

Worse from:
Warmth.
Heat of the bed.

Better for:
Cold applications.

Lycopodium

- Symptoms have a marked tendency to move from right to left.

- Lots of digestive disturbance: belching, rumbling, gurgling, and bloating.

- Marked aggravation between 4–8pm.

- Generally chilly and better for warmth, except for head symptoms which are better from cold.

- Throat symptoms relieved by warm drinks.

- Periodical headaches associated with digestive disturbance.

- Tendency to diarrhoea often combined with anxiety.

- Burning pains especially in the digestive tract.

Worse from:
Late afternoon.
Cold drinks.
Cold air.
Over-exertion.

Better for:
Warmth.
Warm drinks.
Open air.

Mercurius solubilis

- Discharges which are copious and offensive.

- Marked swelling and flabbiness of tongue which takes imprint of teeth.

- Saliva much increased and has metallic taste.

- Tendency to glandular swelling and aching.

- Night sweats very marked with offensive odour.

- Marked tendency for the production of ulcers, abscesses, boils, and pus formation in general.

- Terrific sensitivity to extremes of temperature.

- Most symptoms feel worse from becoming warm in bed.

Worse from:
Night.
Sweating.
Heat of the bed.
Extreme changes of temperature.

Better for:
Resting.
Moderate temperatures.

Natrum mur

Dryness of mucous membranes.

- Nasal discharge alternates between copious, clear mucus, and a thicker, more scanty discharge like egg white.

- Stubborn constipation.

- Skin is generally cracked and dry, especially around the lips.

- Chronic tendency to cold sores.

- Marked emotional disturbance which cannot be released.

- Desire to cry, but cannot, especially in company.

- Symptoms may follow on from suppressed reactions to grief, or reprimand.

- Lots of allergic symptoms: itching skin, sneezing, watery eyes, etc.

Worse from:
Consolation.
Noise.
Talking.

Better for:
Being left alone.
Skipping meals.
Open air.

Nux vomica

- Oversensitivity is marked on both mental and physical levels.

- Often indicated for symptoms which follow 'burning the candle at both ends' or general over-indulgence in food and alcohol.

- Headaches accompany most symptoms: especially constipation.

- With constipation there is a marked symptom of incomplete evacuation of stool with a sensation as though something had been left behind.

- May feel relief would be obtained by vomiting, but must strain to do it.

- Generally very chilly, and feel much worse for being exposed to draughts of cold air.

- Very irritable, snappy, and argumentative.

- Generally much better for being left alone.

Worse from:
Being spoken to.
Any form of stimulation.
Eating.
Being exposed to a chilly, draughty environment.

Better for:
Having a nap.
Being left undisturbed.
Avoiding food.

Phosphorus

- Marked tendency to glandular swellings, and recurrent sore throats.

- Tightness and oppression of chest with irritating, tickly coughs.

- Catarrh is often coloured yellow.

- Hoarseness which gets worse as the evening goes on.

- General tendency to flushes of heat.

- Market thirst for cold drinks.

- Terrific sensitivity to atmospheric changes, e.g. headaches may warn of an approaching thunderstorm.

- Very mentally and physically reactive to stimuli.

- Easily exhausted.

Worse from:
Physical or mental exertion.
In the evening.
Warm food or drink.
In a thunderstorm.

Better for:
Cold food and drink until it gets warmed in the stomach.
Being touched and reassured.

Pulsatilla

- Very chilly but feel much better for fresh, open air.

- Often indicated in the later, established stage of illness.

- Changeability of symptoms on both emotional and physical levels.

- Discharges from mucus membranes may be thick, green and bland.

- Weepiness accompanies most symptoms with a strong need for sympathy.

- Dry mouth with no thirst.

- Sensitivity to rich and fatty foods which leads to indigestion.

Worse from:
Stuffy rooms.
Resting.
After eating.

Better for:
Gentle exercise.
Open, fresh air.
Sympathy.

Rhus tox

- Aching limbs and joints that are relieved from gentle exercise, but feel worse from over-exertion.

- Most symptoms are much worse at night, especially in bed.

- Very sensitive to cold and damp.

- Pains are relieved by a warm bath.

- Very restless and despondent with pain.

- Aching in bones with fevers and influenza.

- Skin can be intolerably itchy, red and blistered.

Worse from:
Keeping still.
Over-exertion.
Cold, wet weather.
At night.

Better for:
Gentle movement.
Warmth.
Dry weather.

Homoeopathic remedies and their abbreviations

Remedy	Abbreviated name
Aconitum napelus	Aconite
Aesculus hippocastanum	Aesculus
Allium cepa	
Alumina	
Antimonium crudum	Antimonium crud
Antimonium tartaricum	Antimonium tart
Apis mellifica	Apis
Arnica montana	Arnica
Arsenicum album	Arsenicum alb
Belladonna	
Bryonia alba	Bryonia
Calcarea carbonica	Calc carb
Calcarea phosphorica	Calc phos
Calendula officinalis	Calendula

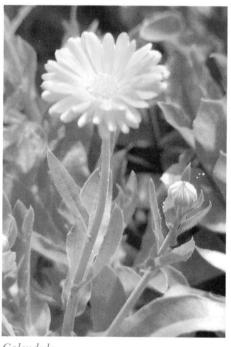

Calendula

Cantharis	
Carbo vegetabilis	Carbo veg

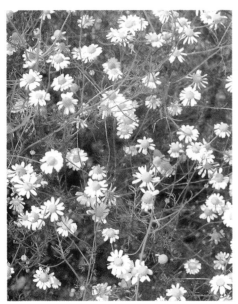

Chamomilla

Chamomilla	
Colocynthis	
Cuprum metallicum	Cuprum
Dulcamara	
Eupatorium perfoliatum	Eupatorium
Euphrasia	
Ferrum metallicum	Ferrum met
Ferrum phosphoricum	Ferrum phos
Gelsemium sempervirens	Gelsemium
Glonoine	
Hamamelis virginica	Hamamelis
Hepar sulphuris calcareum	Hepar sulph
Hypericum perfoliatum	Hypericum
Ignatia amara	Ignatia
Ipecacuana	Ipecac
Kali bichromium	Kali bich
Kali carbonicum	Kali carb
Ledum palustre	Ledum
Lycopodium	
Mercurius solubilis	Mercurius
Natrum muriaticum	Natrum mur
Nux vomica	Nux vom
Phosphorous	
Phytolacca decandra	Phytolacca
Pulsatilla nigricans	Pulsatilla
Pygrogenium	Pyrogen
Rhus toxicodendron	Rhus tox
Rumex crispus	Rumex

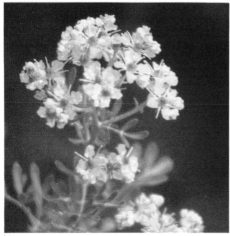

Ruta

Ruta graveolens   Ruta
Sanguinaria
Sepia
Silica
Spongia tosta   Spongia
Sulphur   Sulph
Symphytum officinale   Symphytum

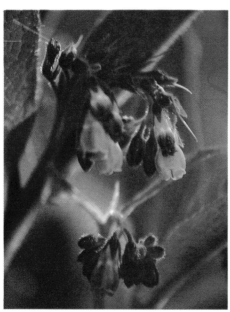

Symphytum

Thuja occidentalis   Thuja
Urtica urens   Urtica
Veratrum album   Veratrum alb

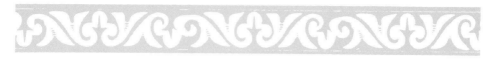

FURTHER READING

Specific books on self-help

The Complete Homoeopathy Handbook: A Guide to Everyday Health Care,
Miranda Castro; Macmillan, 1990.
*Everybody's Guide to Homoeopathic Medicines: Taking Care of Yourself and Your
Family with Safe and Effective Remedies*, Stephen Cummings and Dana
Ullmann; Gollancz, 1986.
How To Use Homoeopathy, Dr Christopher Hammond; Element, 1991.
The Family Guide to Homoeopathy: The Safe Form of Medicine for the Future,
Dr Andrew Lockie; Elm Tree Books, 1989.
Homoeopathic Medicine at Home, Maesimund Panof and Jane Heimlich;
Corgi, 1980.

General introductions to homoeopathy

New Ways To Health, A Guide to Homoeopathy, Sarah Richardson; Hamlyn,
1988.
Homoeopathy, Medicine for the 21st Century, Dana Ullmann; North Atlantic
Books, 1988.
Homoeopathy, Medicine for the New Man, George Vithoulkas; Thorsons,
London.
The Complete Book of Homoeopathy, Michael Weiner and Kathleen Goss;
Bantam, 1982.

If you wish to go beyond a general introduction to homoeopathy and
obtain more specific information on the theory and philosophy of
homoeopathy as a medical science, the following books will be of interest:

*Homoeopathic Science and Modern Medicine: The Physics of Healing With
Microdoses*, Harris Coulter; North Atlantic Books, 1980.
The Science of Homoeopathy, George Vithoulkas; Thorsons, London.

Books which provide an overview of the historical development of
homoeopathy include:

The Two Faces of Homoeopathy, Anthony Campbell; Robert Hale Ltd.,
London, 1984.
*Divided Legacy: The Conflict Between Homoeopathy and the American Medical
Association*, Harris Coulter; North Atlantic Books, 1982.
Homoeopathy and the Medical Profession, Phillip Nicholls; Croom Helm,
1988.

Vaccination

The following provide a survey of the arguments for and against immunisation:

Vaccination and Immunization: Dangers, Delusions and Alternatives, Leon Chaitow; C W Daniel, 1987.
Vaccination, A Difficult Decision, a leaflet published by the Society of Homoeopaths, Felicity Lee; September 1991.
The Immunization Decision: A Guide for Parents, Dr Randall Neustaedter; North Atlantic Books, 1990.

Veterinary homoeopathy

The Homoeopathic Treatment of Small Animals, Principles and Practice, Christopher Day; Wigmore Publications Ltd., 1984.
Cats: Homoeopathic Remedies, George MacLeod; C W Daniel, 1990.
Dogs: Homoeopathic Remedies, George MacLeod; C W Daniel, 1983.

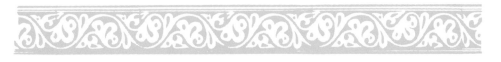

USEFUL ADDRESSES

British Homoeopathic Association
27a Devonshire Street
London
W1N 1RJ

The Society of Homoeopaths
2 Artizan Road
Northampton
NN1 4HU

The Hahnemann Society
Humane Education Centre
Avenue Lodge
Bounds Green Road
London
NE22 4EU

Homoeopathic Development
Foundation Ltd.
Harcourt House
19a Cavendish Square
London
W1M 9AD

Council for Complementary and
Alternative Medicine
Suite 1
19a Cavendish Square
London
W1M 9AD

Institute for Complementary
Medicine
Unit 4
Tavern Quay
Rope Street
Rotherhithe
London
SE16

Natural Medicines Society
Edith Lewis House
Back Lane
Ilkeston
Derbyshire
DE7 8EJ

How and where to train as a homoeopath

The following list includes many of the colleges which offer courses in homoeopathy. A more comprehensive list may be obtained from the Society of Homoeopaths.

Faculty of Homoeopathy
Royal London Homoeopathic
Hospital
Great Ormond Street
London
WC1N 3HR

Midlands College of Homoeopathy
186 Wolverhampton Street
Dudley
West Midlands
DY1 3AD

College of Homoeopathy
26 Clarendon Rise
London
SE13 6JR

London College of Classical
Homoeopathy
63 Maycross Avenue
Morden
Surrey

Northern College of
Homoeopathic Medicine
First Floor
Swinburne House
Swinburne Street
Gateshead
Tyne and Wear
NE8 1AX

The Small School of Homoeopathy
Out of the Blue Centre
North Street
Cromford
Derbyshire
DE4 3RG

Homoeopathic Hospitals

The Royal London Homoeopathic
Hospital
Great Ormond Street
London
WC1N 3HR

Glasgow Homoeopathic Hospital
100 Great Western Road
Glasgow
G12 0RN

Bristol Homoeopathic Hospital
Cotham Road
Cotham
Bristol
BS6 6UJ

Tunbridge Wells Homoeopathic
Hospital
Church Road
Tunbridge Wells
Kent
TN1 1JU

Department of Homoeopathic
Medicine
Mossley Hill Hospital
Park Avenue
Liverpool
L18 8BU

Homoeopathic pharmacies and suppliers

Ainsworths
38 New Cavendish Street
London
W1M 7LH

Galen Pharmacy
1 South Street
Dorchester
Dorset
DT1 1DE

Helios
92 Camden Road
Tunbridge Wells
Kent
TN1 2QP

Nelson's Pharmacies Limited
73 Duke Street
London
W1M 6BY

Weleda UK Limited
Heanor Road
Ilkeston
Derbyshire
DE7 8DR

Boxes for storing remedies, phials and other homoeopathic supplies can
be obtained from:

The Homoeopathic Supply Company
4 Nelson Road
Sherringham
Norfolk
NR26 8BU